CORONARY TONE IN ISCHEMIC HEART DISEASE

DEVELOPMENTS IN CARDIOVASCULAR MEDICINE

Lancée CT, ed: Echocardiology, 1979. ISBN 90-247-2209-8.

Baan J, Arntzenius AC, Yellin EL, eds: Cardiac dynamics. 1980. ISBN 90-247-2212-8.

Thalen HJT, Meere CC, eds: Fundamentals of cardiac pacing. 1970. ISBN 90-247-2245-4.

Kulbertus HE, Wellens HJJ, eds: Sudden death. 1980. ISBN 90-247-2290-X.

Dreifus LS, Brest AN, eds: Clinical applications of cardiovascular drugs. 1980. ISBN 90-247-2295-0.

Spencer MP, Reid JM, eds: Cerebrovascular evaluation with Doppler ultrasound. 1981. ISBN 90-247-2348-1.

Zipes DP, Bailey JC, Elharrar V, eds: The slow inward current and cardiac arrhythmias. 1980. ISBN 90-247-2380-9.

Kesteloot H, Joossens JV, eds: Epidemiology of arterial blood pressure. 1980. ISBN 90-247-2386-8.

Wackers FJT, ed: Thallium-201 and technetium-99m-pyrophosphate myocardial imaging in the coronary care unit.
1980. ISBN 90-247-2396-5.

Maseri A, Marchesi C, Chierchia S, Trivella MG, eds: Coronary care units. 1981. ISBN 90-247-2456-2.

Morganroth J, Moore EN, Dreifus LS, Michelson EL, eds: The evaluation of new antiarrhythmic drugs. 1981.
ISBN 90-247-2474-0.

Alboni P: Intraventricular conduction disturbances. 1981. ISBN 90-247-2484-X.

Rijsterborgh H, ed: Echocardiology. 1981. ISBN 90-247-2491-0.

Wagner GS, ed: Myocardial infarction: Measurement and intervention. 1982. ISBN 90-247-2513-5.

Meltzer RS, Roelandt J, eds: Contrast echocardiography. 1982. ISBN 90-247-2531-3.

Amery A, Fagard R, Lijnen R, Staessen J, eds: Hypertensive cardiovascular disease; pathophysiology and treatment.
1982. ISBN 90-247-2534-8.

Bouman LN, Jongsma HJ, eds: Cardiac rate and rhythm. 1982. ISBN 90-247-2626-3.

Morganroth J, Moore EN, eds: The evaluation of beta blocker and calcium antagonist drugs. 1982.
ISBN 90-247-2642-5.

Rosenbaum MB, ed: Frontiers of cardiac electrophysiology. 1982. ISBN 90-247-2663-8.

Roelandt J, Hugenholtz PG, eds: Long-term ambulatory electrocardiography. 1982. ISBN 90-247-2664-8.

Adgey AAJ, ed: Acute phase of ischemic heart disease and myocardial infarction. 1982. ISBN 90-247-2675-1.

Hanrath P, Bleifeld W, Souquet, J. eds: Cardiovascular diagnosis by ultrasound. Transesophageal, computerized,
contrast, Doppler echocardiography. 1982. ISBN 90-247-2692-1.

Roelandt J, ed: The practice of M-mode and two-dimensional echocardiography. 1983. ISBN 90-247-2745-6.

Meyer J, Schweizer P, Erbel R, eds: Advances in noninvasive cardiology. 1983. ISBN 0-89838-576-8.

Morganroth J, Moore EN, eds: Sudden cardiac death and congestive heart failure: Diagnosis and treatment. 1983.
ISBN 0-89838-580-6.

Perry HM, ed: Lifelong management of hypertension. 1983. ISBN 0-89838-582-2.

Jaffe EA, ed: Biology of endothelial cells. 1984. ISBN 0-89838-587-3.

Surawicz B, Reddy CP, Prystowsky EN, eds: Tachycardias. ISBN 0-89838-588-1.

Spencer MP, ed: Cardiac Doppler diagnosis. 1983. ISBN 0-89838-591-1.

Villarreal H, Sambhi MP, eds: Topics in pathophysiology of hypertension. 1984. ISBN 0-89838-595-4.

Messerli FH, ed: Cardiovascular disease in the elderly. 1984. ISBN 0-89838-596-2.

Simoons ML, Reiber JHC, eds: Nuclear imaging in clinical cardiology. 1984. ISBN 0-89838-599-7.

Ter Keurs HEDJ, Schipperheyn JJ, eds: Cardiac left ventricular hypertrophy. 1983. ISBN 0-89838-612-8.

Sperelakis N, ed: Physiology and pathophysiology of the heart. ISBN 0-89838-612-2.

Messerli FH, ed: Kidney in essential hypertension. ISBN 0-89838-616-0.

Sambhi MP, ed: Fundamental fault in hypertension. ISBN 0-89838-638-1.

Marchesi C, ed: Ambulatory monitoring: Cardiovascular system and allied applications. ISBN 0-89838-642-X.

Kupper W, MacAlpin RN, Bleifeld W, eds: Coronary tone in ischemic heart disease. ISBN 0-89838-646-2.

Sperelakis N, Caulfield JB, eds: Calcium antagonists: Mechanisms of action on cardiac muscle and vascular smooth
muscle. ISBN 0-89838-655-1.

Godfraind T, Herman AS, Wellens D, eds: Calcium entry blockers in cardiovascular and cerebral dysfunctions.
ISBN 0-89838-658-1.

Morganroth J, Moore EN, eds: Interventions in the acute phase of myocardial infarction. ISBN 0-89838-659-4.

CORONARY TONE IN ISCHEMIC HEART DISEASE

edited by

WOLFRAM KUPPER, MD
Department of Cardiology, University Hospital Hamburg, Eppendorf, FRG

REX N. MacALPIN, MD
Department of Cardiology, University of California, Los Angeles, USA

WALTER BLEIFELD, MD
Department of Cardiology, University Hospital Hamburg, Eppendorf, FRG

1984 **MARTINUS NIJHOFF PUBLISHERS**
a member of the KLUWER ACADEMIC PUBLISHERS GROUP
BOSTON / DORDRECHT / LANCASTER

Distributors

for the United States and Canada: Kluwer Academic Publishers, 190 Old Derby Street, Hingham, MA 02043, USA
for the UK and Ireland: Kluwer Academic Publishers, MTP Press Limited, Falcon House, Queen Square, Lancaster LA1 1RN, England
for all other countries: Kluwer Academic Publishers Group, Distribution Center, P.O. Box 322, 3300 AH Dordrecht, The Netherlands

Library of Congress Cataloging in Publication Data

```
Coronary tone in ischemic heart disease.

  (Developments in cardiovascular medicine)
  Includes bibliographical references and index.
  1. Coronary vasospasm.  2. Coronary arteries--Effect
of drugs on.  3. Vasodilators.  I. Kupper, Wolfram.
II. MacAlpin, Rex N.  III. Bleifeld, W. (Walter)
IV. Series.  [DNLM: 1. Coronary vasospasm--Etiology.
2. Coronary vasospasm--Drug effects.  3. Coronary
vessels--Pathology.  W1 DE997VME / WG 300 C8257]
RC685.C65C684  1984      616.1'23      84-4130
ISBN 0-89838-646-2
```

Table of contents

Acknowledgments   VII

List of contributors   IX

1.   Introduction
     W. Kupper   1

2.   Relation of coronary arterial spasm to sites of organic stenosis
     R.N. MacAlpin   5

3.   The concept of dynamic coronary stenoses
     W. Rafflenbeul   19

4.   Contribution of dynamic vascular wall thickening to luminal narrow-
     ing during coronary arterial vasomotion
     P.W. Serruys, J.M. Lablanche, J.W. Deckers, J.H.C. Reiber, M.W.
     Bertrand & P.G. Hugenholtz   25

5.   Alteration in coronary vasomotor tone by alpha-stimulation
     E. Bassenge & J. Holtz   43

6.   Regulation of large coronary arteries by beta adrenergic mechanisms
     in conscious dogs
     S.F. Vatner & T.H. Hintze   57

7.   The role of alpha-adrenergic activity in large and small coronary
     arteries in man
     M. Mishima, M. Inoue, M. Hori, T. Shimazu, H. Abe, K. Kodama &
     S. Nanto   75

8.   Adrenergic control of human coronary circulation
     G.H. Mudge, Jr. & P. Ganz   89

9.   The effect of cardioselective beta blockade by metoprolol on the
     coronary vascular tone under endogenous catecholamine stimulation
     C.W. Hamm, A. Deppe, W. Bleifeld & W. Kupper   95

VI

10. Alpha-adrenergic receptors and coronary vasospasm
     S. Chierchia   105

11. Enhanced transcardiac 1-norepinephrine response during cold pres-
     sor test in obstructive coronary artery disease
     H.S. Mueller, P.S. Rao, P.B. Rao, D.J. Gory & S.M. Ayres   115

Subject index   127

Acknowledgments

All papers and discussions in this book were presented at a workshop in April 22nd, 1983 in Lübeck-Travemünde, FRG during the annual meeting of the European Society for Clinical Investigation (ESCI). We would like to express our thanks to the authorities of the ESCI, especially to the local organizers Prof. H. Greten and Prof. G. Klose of the Department of Medicine, University Hospital Hamburg, for initiating this meeting.

The workshop was found to be very fruitful for the exchange of information and ideas between specialists in various cardiovascular disciplines in a pleasant and lively atmosphere.

We are indebted to Mr. B. Commandeur from Martinus Nijhoff Publishers for his valuable support and advice.

The editors

List of contributors

Bassenge, E., Albrecht-Ludwigs-Universität, Lehrstuhl für Angewandte Physiologie, Hermann-Herder-Strasse 7, D-7800 Freiburg, FRG
co-author: J. Holtz

Chierchia, S., University of London, Royal Postgraduate Medical School, Hammersmith Hospital, Ducane Road, London W12 0HS, UK

Hamm, C.W., Universitäts Krankenhaus Eppendorf, Medizinische Klinik II, Martinistrasse 52, D-2000 Hamburg, FRG
co-authors: A. Deppe, W. Bleifeld, W. Kupper

MacAlpin, R.N., Department of Medicine, UCLA School of Medicine, UCLA Center for the Health Sciences, Los Angeles, CA 90024, USA

Mishima, M., The First Department of Medicine, Osaka University School of Medicine, 1-1-50 Fukushima, Fukushima-ku, Osaka 553, Japan
co-authors: M. Inoue, M. Hori, T. Shimazu, H. Abe (The First Department of Medicine, Osaka University School of Medicine, Osaka, Japan), K. Kodama, S. Nanto (Cardiac Intensive Care Unit, Osaka Police Hospital, Osaka, Japan)

Mudge, G.H., Jr., Harvard Medical School, Clinical Cardiology Service, Brigham and Women's Hospital, Boston, MA 02115, USA
co-author: P. Ganz

Mueller, H.S., Division of Cardiology, Montefiore Medical Center, 111 East 210th Street, Bronx, NY 10467, USA
co-authors: P.S. Rao, P.B. Rao, D.J. Gory, S.M. Ayres

Rafflenbeul, W., Medizinische Hochschule Hannover, Abteilung Kardiologie, Zentrum für Innere Medizin und Dermatologie, Postfach 610180, D-3000 Hannover 61, FRG

Serruys, P.W., Catheterization Laboratory, Thoraxcenter, Erasmus University, P.O. Box 1738, 3000 DR Rotterdam, The Netherlands
co-authors: J.M. Lablanche, J.W. Deckers, J.H.C. Reiber, M.E. Bertrand (Hôpital Cardiologique, Lille, France)

Vatner, S.F., New England Regional Primate Research Center, 1 Pine Hill Drive, Southbore, MA 01772, USA
co-author: T.H. Hintze

1. Introduction

W. KUPPER

Coronary artery vasoconstriction is not only the mechanism responsible for Prinzmetal's variant angina, but may also be involved in stable angina pectoris and myocardial infarction. However, the underlying patho-physiological mechanisms and the importance of coronary vasoconstriction in these syndromes is still largely unknown. Several hypotheses have been proposed. Sympathetic nervous activity plays a key role in the regulation of coronary blood flow, but mechanical or humoral constrictive factors may be active as well.

α-adrenergic tone

Adrenergic nerve fibers accompany coronary vessels of any size. The stimulation of cardiac sympathetic nerves causes an increase in coronary blood flow. If, however, chronotropic and inotropic effects of adrenergic stimulation are suppressed pharmacologically by beta-adrenoceptor blockade, a reduction in flow is observed. Thus, the primary effect of sympathetic stimulation on the coronary arteries is the alpha-adrenergic mediated vasoconstriction. Functionally innervated alpha-adrenoceptors have been documented both in large coronary conductance arteries and in the small resistance vessels. Animal studies and a human study have documented that a permanent constrictor tone is present on the coronary circulation both at rest and during exercise; this condition could be prevented with alpha-adrenoceptor blockade or was absent after heart transplantation. Therefore, alpha-adrenoceptor mediated coronary constriction is an attractive hypothesis as a possible pathophysiological mechanism of inappropriate coronary vasoconstriction and coronary vasospasm. This concept was supported by the finding of an exercise induced coronary vasospasm and the occurrence of transient ST-segment elevation in patients with variant angina after injection of Epinephrine and occasionally after exposure to cold. Alpha-adrenoceptor blockade with Phentolamine and Phenoxybenzamine prevented these effects.

Intensive studies of sympathetic function in patients with Prinzmetal's angina, however, revealed no apparent resting abnormality compared with patients without chest pain. Furthermore, plasma catecholamine levels were not in-

Kupper, W. (ed.), Coronary tone in ischemic heart disease. ISBN 0-89838-646-2.
© *1984, Martinus Nijhoff Publishers, Boston/The Hague/Dordrecht/Lancaster. Printed in the Netherlands.*

creased at the onset of the attacks. Recently, several clinical trials with different kinds of pharmacologically alpha-adrenoceptor blockade have failed to demonstrate a positive effect on patients with vasospastic angina. So, at present, it is still open to question whether or not the alpha-adrenergic system is the physiologic mediator of an inappropriate coronary artery vasoconstriction. It seems rather unlikely, that a general increase in sympathetic outflow to the heart itself can initiate coronary spasm. The role of alpha-adrenergic receptors in the pathogenesis of coronary artery spasm must continue to be questioned.

β-adrenergic tone

Beta adrenoceptor activation elicits an increase in coronary blood flow even if myocardial metabolic demands are held constant. The isoproterenol induced vasodilation was thought to be primarily mediated by stimulation of vascular beta$_2$-receptors in coronary resistance vessels. Recently it has been demonstrated in the conscious dog that isoproterenol also directly increases the cross sectional area of large coronary arteries. Furthermore it was shown that this effect occured not only in response to beta$_2$-adrenergic receptor stimulation, or an increase in myocardial metabolic demand, but also in response to direct stimulation of beta$_2$ vascular adrenergic receptors.

Propranolol blocks beta$_1$ and beta$_2$ adrenergic receptors and induces a modest constriction of large coronary arteries in the conscious dog. Is this mediated by inhibition of beta-adrenergic tone and changes in myocardial metabolic demands or due to the response of unopposed alpha-adrenergic tone? Evidence suggests that the latter is more unlikely. In the conscious animal it has not been possible to induce spasm of an epicardial coronary artery by any means of pharmacological beta-adrenoceptor blockade irrespective of whether beta$_1$, beta$_2$ or both receptor types were blocked. This was also true after additional alpha-adrenoceptor stimulation.

In view of these results it was necessary to investigate the potential role of beta-adrenergic mechanisms mediating vasospasm of large coronary arteries in man, since beta-adrenergic blockade with propranolol has been reported to intensify the duration as well as the degree of myocardial ischemia in patients with a history of coronary artery spasm. The mechanism, by which the exacerbation of vasospastic angina is mediated, has not been completely elucidated but seems to be a dose-dependent phenomenon. In high doses of up to 1 g/24 h, an earlier study reported beneficial effects. On the other hand it has been shown that acute intravenous beta-adrenergic blockade can increase the adrenergically mediated vasoconstrictor response in terms of coronary vascular resistance to the cold pressor test in conditions of exhausted coronary reserve.

It has to be assumed that all of the experimental studies mentioned above were carried out with pharmacological activation or blockade of adrenergic receptors.

Thus, the role of beta-adrenergic receptor regulation of large coronary arteries by neural activation remains to be demonstrated. Furthermore, it is extremely difficult to get an experimental set up which can distinguish the primary effect of nervous control of coronary arteries from the secondary effect brought about by the simultaneous change in heart work. Presently we cannot exclude the possibility that beta-adrenoceptor blockade with a non-selective beta-blocker aggravates episodes of vasospastic angina in some patients by an as yet unknown mechanism. However, it is known that sympathetic nervous activity may enhance ventricular irritability and lower the threshold to ventricular fibrillation in the ischemic myocardium. This mechanism could increase the risk of the patient with coronary artery disease, and the author supports the view that reducing overall sympathetic tone by anti-adrenergic agents might be a useful therapeutic intervention for patients with ischemic heart disease.

Humoral and mechanical factors

Atherosclerotic altered regions of large coronary arteries are prone to changes in vasomotor reactivity. The arteries of patients with inappropriate vasomotor tone are especially sensitive to ergonovine at the sites of the arteriosclerotic lesions. Therefore, hyper reactivity occurs rather locally and not uniformly. The hypersensitivity of arteriosclerotic arteries to ergonovine was recently attributed to a serotoninergic mechanism, which could not be inhibited by alpha-adrenergic blockers. Unfortunately the first experiences with serotonin antagonists like ketanserin failed to prevent ergonovine induced myocardial ischemia in patients with vasospastic angina.

Another important aspect is that the diameter of large coronary arteries is influenced by changes in coronary artery blood flow. The reactive dilatation of these arteries after brief periods of occlusion can be prevented by suppression of reactive hyperemia. This result supports the hypothesis that neurogenic constrictor influences on epicardial vessels may be effectively counteracted by endothelium mediated, flow-dependent dilatation, which serves as a protective mechanism against all kinds of constrictive stimuli. If this protective mechanism is lost by localized endothelial damage or low coronary flow, vasoconstriction may occur. This hypothesis in man has yet to be confirmed. The only substantial evidence is that a coronary vasospasm occurs locally, preferably at night, shows cyclic variations with active and quiescent phases and up to now has never been described in children.

All of these questions are extensively discussed in the following chapters in order to give an up-to-date overview of the current trends in this rapidly developing field of cardiovascular medicine.

2. Relation of coronary arterial spasm to sites of organic stenosis

REX N. MACALPIN

Coronary arterial spasm is a problem of older adults; it has not to my knowledge been described in children. This suggests that a prerequisite is a coronary artery which has acquired an abnormality as it has aged. Variant angina is a condition most commonly due to large coronary artery spasm. In the 80 patients I have personally seen with it, angiographically detectable disease was present in the vessel involved with spasm in 95% of cases. Careful study of cases presented in the literature as having 'normal' coronary arteries actually reveals in many instances minor, persistent irregularities in the vessel which goes into spasm.

Several years ago I reviewed then available information on the relation of coronary spasm to specific sites of organic stenosis [1]. Combining my own experience with that published by others, I found 137 cases of variant angina where spontaneous or ergonovine-induced coronary spasm causing myocardial ischemia was documented angiographically. One hundred twelve (82%) of these had some organic disease noted. Of these 112 cases there were 104 in whom the coronary spasm involved only one vessel, and 99 of these (95%) had angiographically detectable disease in that vessel.

These 104 cases of single vessel coronary spasm are graphically shown in Figure 1. Several observations can be made from this figure. There was a high incidence of essentially single vessel organic disease with 70 cases (67%) having only one coronary artery narrowed more than 10% of its diameter. There was also a relatively uniform distribution of the degree of organic stenosis in the 'spastic' artery, ranging from minimal disease to severe luminal obstruction. Coronary spasm occurred in the most severely diseased vessel in 67 cases (64%). However, in about 10% of cases the spasm occurred in a vessel with little or no discernible disease. When each of two vessels was significantly narrowed, the degree of stenosis was not a reliable guide to which underwent spasm, unless the 'non-spastic' vessel was occluded.

I next looked for cases of coronary spasm in which there was a description of the precise location of the spasm in relation to the existing organic disease. Sixty-nine cases were found (nine personally observed and 60 published by others). In 62 of these (90%) the spasm causing ischemia was precisely superimposed on and limited to the site of the preexisting organic lesion (admittedly the distal limit of

Kupper, W. (ed.), Coronary tone in ischemic heart disease. ISBN 0-89838-646-2.
© 1984, Martinus Nijhoff Publishers, Boston/The Hague/Dordrecht/Lancaster. Printed in the Netherlands.

6

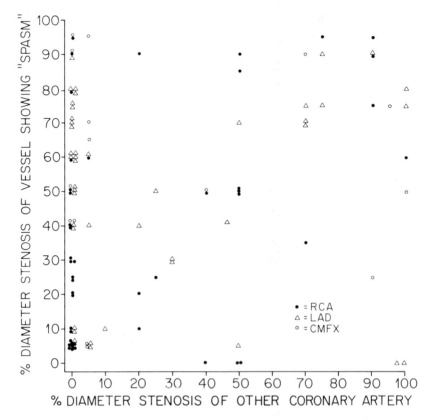

Figure 1. Percent organic diameter stenosis found between attacks in the coronary artery manifesting spasm during an anginal attack in 104 patients with vasotonic angina (vertical axis) correlated with the degree of organic stenosis present in the same cases in the next most severely diseased but 'nonspastic' coronary artery (horizontal axis). Solid circles, open triangles and open circles identify the specific 'spastic' vessel, which is, respectively, the right coronary artery (RCA), the anterior descending artery (LAD), and the left circumflex coronary artery (CMFX). Lesions described only as 'plaques' have arbitrarily been assigned a magnitude of 5% diameter stenosis (reprinted from Am J Cardiol 46:143, 1980, with permission).

the spasm was frequently indeterminate when spasm occluded the vessel). In four cases the spasm seemed centered in an area of vessel with the organic lesions, but extended over a 2–4-cm length of the vessel, involving some sections that had previously appeared normal. In one case spasm occurred at the site of a high grade organic lesion, but occurred simultaneously at a focal site in an apparently normal portion of the distal vessel. In only two cases did severe spasm occur exclusively in apparently normal portions of a coronary artery that contained organic stenoses themselves uninvolved with spasm.

Of 51 autopsied cases of variant angina reported in the literature, 45 (88%) revealed organic coronary disease in the vessel in whose distribution the transient ST segment elevation occurred: in two cases there were equivocal abnormalities,

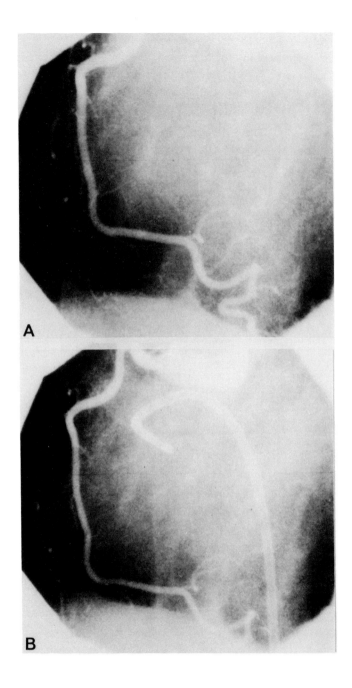

Figure 2. Two frames from a coronary cinearteriographic stufy of the right coronary artery of a 62-year-old woman without coronary disease. Left anterior oblique projection: A. before drugs; B. after 0.4 mg ergonovine maleate i.v.

8

and in only four cases were the arteries said to be histologically normal.

Sixteen cases were found in the literature in which histologic examination was made of the segment of coronary artery previously shown to undergo ischemia-provoking spasm by arteriography. The coronary segments were removed at surgery in seven cases [2–4], and studied at autopsy in the other nine cases [5–11]. In 15 cases there was some organic disease present in the segment susceptible to

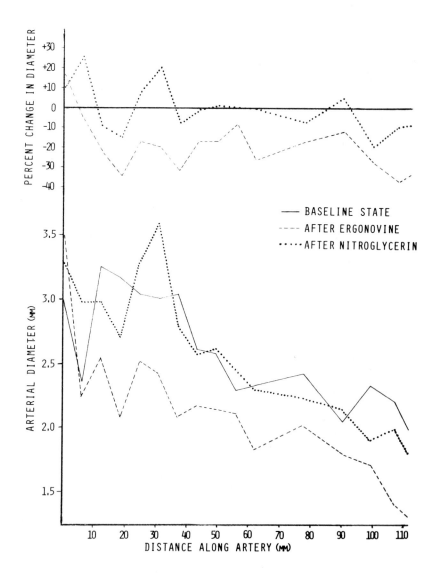

Figure 3. Measurements of coronary arterial diameter taken from images shown in Figure 2 at matched points along the vessel. Nitroglycerin 0.1 mg was given i.v. after ergonovine effect was recorded (post nitroglycerin image not shown in Figure 2).

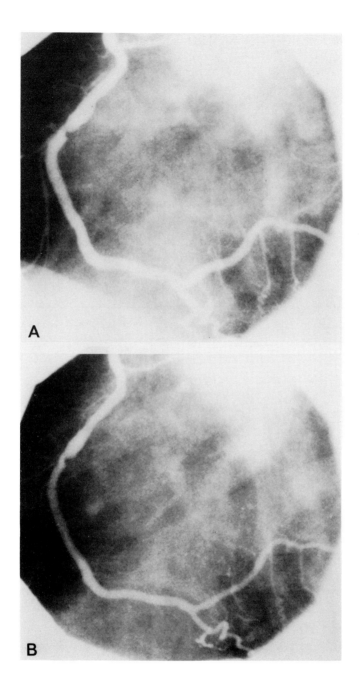

Figure 4. Frames from a coronary cinearteriographic study of the right coronary artery in a 55-year-old man with classic coronary heart disease. Left anterior oblique projection: A. before drugs; B. after 0.4 mg ergonovine maleate i.v.

10

spasm. In one case the spasm was said to have occluded the vessel 1 cm proximal to a 90% diameter stenosis, but the presence or absence of histologic disease at this point was not commented on [9]; the vessel was, however, not arteriographically normal at this point between anginal attacks. In three cases the coronary disease was believed to be nonatheromatous [2, 6]. This group of sixteen cases is, of course, biased to include a large proportion of cases with more

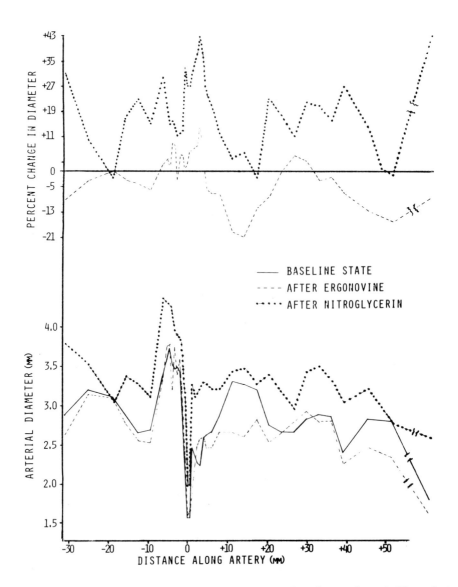

Figure 5. Measurements of coronary arterial diameter taken from images shown in Figure 4 at matched points along the vessel. Nitroglycerin 0.3 mg was given i.v. after ergonovine effect was recorded. Post nitroglycerin image not shown in Figure 4.

severe organic disease, which accounted for the surgical treatment allowing the biopsy, and which is correlated with a higher mortality risk [12].

It has been known for years that disease of the coronary arteries can alter their vasomotor reactivity. Some interesting observations can be made by careful quantitation of the responses of long arterial segments to vaso-active stimuli in vivo. Figure 2 shows frames from a 35-mm coronary cine-angiographic study of a 62-year-old woman with atypical, noncardiac, chest pain. Views of the right coronary artery from the same part of the cardiac cycle are shown with identical magnification before drugs were given (Figure 2A), and after ergonovine maleate in total dose of 0.4 mg (Figure 2B). Careful measurements from these images were made at identical sites along the vessel in the different states, and these are presented graphically in Figure 3. Ergonovine produced a constriction of the artery which was fairly *uniform* along its length, except near the origin where mild catheter induced spasm had occurred before drugs were given. Over most of the vessel the usual post-nitroglycerin arterial dilation compared to the baseline state was not seen, indicating a competition between ergonovine and nitroglycerin. There was a moderate variability of the post-ergonovine nitroglycerin response along the course of the vessel which might be due to early disease of the vascular wall in this patient with coronary arteries deemed normal by the usual ar-teriographic criteria.

In Figures 4 and 5, a similar study is shown of the right coronary artery of a 55-year-old man with classic coronary disease, one month following a small posterior myocardial infarction caused by occlusion of a marginal branch of the left circumflex artery. There was diffuse disease of the right coronary artery; no segment could be clearly called normal, but the worst obstruction was an eccentric diameter stenosis of about 50%. There was marked variability of the vessel's responsiveness to ergonovine along its length and to the subsequently administered nitroglycerin – presumably as a result of disease. The eccentric 50% stenotic lesion was unresponsive to ergonovine, but did dilate significantly after nitroglycerin, suggesting that it might have been in its most constricted state before any drug was given. Had the smooth muscle at the lesion site responded to ergonovine to the same degree as it did in the vessel on either side of the lesion, an important decrease in luminal dimension at the stenosis might have occurred [13].

In Figures 6 and 7, the same type of study is demonstrated in the anterior descending coronary artery of a 60-year-old man with recent onset of effort angina. Treadmill exercise resulted in angina, ST segment elevation in anterior precordial leads, and hypotension. The baseline angiogram showed a 50% diameter stenosis of the anterior descending artery straddling the vessel at the origin of its major diagonal branch. There was marked variability of response to ergonovine only in the immediate vicinity of this lesion. At the stenosis itself there was an exaggerated response to ergonovine which produced a flow-reducing, approximately 85% diameter stenosis accompanied by angina and ST segment elevation in lead V3. The response of the vessel beyond this region, and responses

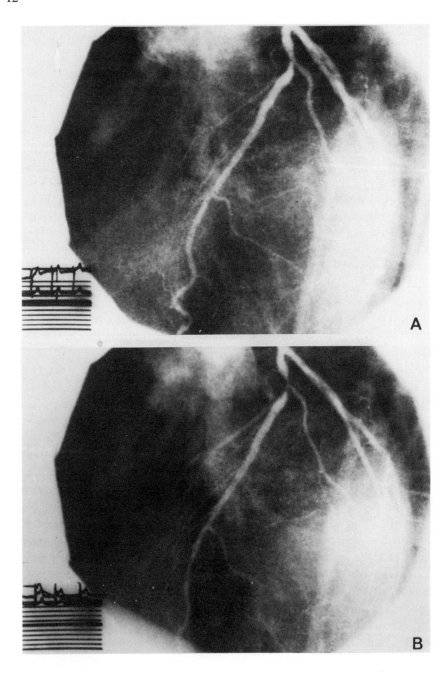

Figure 6. Frames from a coronary cinearteriographic study of the left coronary artery in a 60-year-old man with vasotonic, effort angina. Left anterior oblique projection with cranial angulation: A. before drugs; B. after a total of 0.175 mg ergonovine i.v.; onset of angina and ST segment elevation with slow flow of contrast medium down anterior descending artery.

of other vessels were within the range seen in normal persons. The lesion did not dilate beyond its baseline state after nitroglycerin, possibly because of the competing effect of the ergonovine as seen in the distal parts of the vessel, or because the lesion site was in a state of maximum dilation before drugs were given.

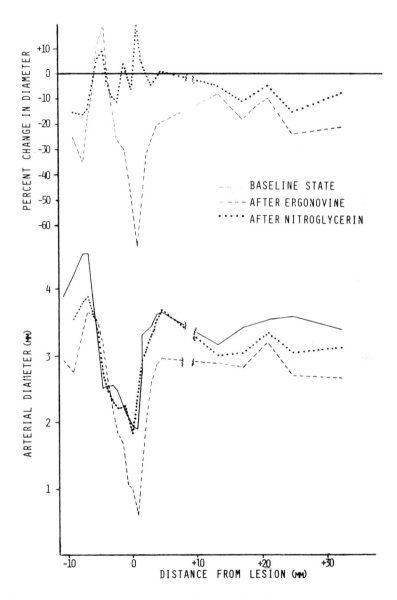

Figure 7. Measurements of coronary arterial diameter taken from images shown in Figure 6 at matched points along the course of the anterior descending vessel. Nitroglycerin 0.2 mg was given i.v. after ergonovine effect was recorded (post nitroglycerin image not shown in Figure 6).

14

Conclusions. Disease of the large coronary arteries usually alters their vasomotor reactivity irregularly and focally rather than uniformly. My overall impression, based on personal observations, is that a generalized vasoconstriction of all major coronary arteries accompanies attacks of vasotonic angina, with the change in luminal diameter usually being within the physiologic range in normal segments of all vessels. Exaggerated focal decrease in luminal size consistent with spasm is usually limited to areas of preexisting organic stenosis, and the transient changes produced in some, but not all, of these lesions are sufficient to produce local myocardial ischemia.

This intimate association of flow-restricting dynamic coronary obstruction and organic arterial lesions is seen in most patients with vasotonic angina, and must be explained by hypotheses which attempt to describe the pathophysiology of coronary arterial spasm.

References

1. MacAlpin RN: Relation of coronary arterial spasm to sites of organic stenosis. Am J Cardiol 46:143–153, 1980.
2. Guermonprez J-L, Gúeret P, Camilleri JP, Gúerinon J, Deloche A, Maurice P: Angor de Prinzmetal. Etude histologique coronaire de prélèvements peropératoires. A propos de deux cas. Arch Mal Coeur 70:301–308, 1977.
3. Brown BG: Coronary vasospasm. Observations linking the clinical spectrum of ischemic heart disease to the dynamic pathology of coronary atherosclerosis. Arch Intern Med 141:716–722, 1981.
4. Heupler F: Oral communication, March 10, 1978.
5. Roberts WC, Curry RC Jr., Isner JM, Waller BF, et al: Sudden death in Prinzmetal's angina with coronary spasm documented by angiography. Analysis of three necropsy patients. Am J Cardiol 50:203–210, 1982.
6. Petitier H, de Lajartre AY, Geslin Ph, Godin JF, Victor J, Crochet D, Dupon H: Dysplasie fibreuse intimale coronaire et angor de Prinzmetal. Arch Mal Coeur 71:1053–1059, 1978.
7. Trevi GP, Thiene G, Benussi P, Marini A, Caobelli A, Frasson F, Ambrosio GB, Dal Palu C: Prinzmetal's variant angina – clinical, angiographic and pathological correlations in two typical cases. Eur J Cardiol 4:319–325, 1976.
8. Rizzon P, Rossi L, Calabrese P. Franchini G, Di Biase M: Angiographic and pathologic correlations in Prinzmetal variant angina. Angiology 29: 486–490, 1978.
9. Maseri A, ĹAbbate A, Baroldi G, Cierchia S, Marzilli M, Ballestra AM, Severi S, Parodi O, Biagini A, Distante A, Pesola A: Coronary vasospasm as a possible cause of myocardial infarction. A conclusion derived from the study of 'preinfarction' angina. N Engl J Med 299:1271–1277, 1978.
10. Dhurandhar RW, Watt DL, Silver MD, Trimble AS, Adelman AG: Prinzmetal's variant form of angina with arteriographic evidence of coronary arterial spasm. Am J Cardiol 30:902–905, 1972.
11. Wojtyna W, Wiese KH, Strauss P, Walter J: Prinzmetal-Phänomen und seltene Koronaranomalie als Infarkt- und Todesursache einer 45 jährigen Patientin. Z Kardiol 71:106–111, 1982.
12. Severi S, Davies G, Maseri A, Marzullo P, L'Abbate A: Long-term prognosis of 'variant' angina with medical treatment. Am J Cardiol 46:226–232, 1980.
13. MacAlpin RN: Contribution of dynamic vascular wall thickening to luminal narrowing during coronary arterial constriction. Circulation 61:296–301, 1980.

Discussion

Dr. McGregor: He is telling us we should use the word 'spasm' more carefully. True spasm of a smooth muscle means an excessive contraction outside the range of normal. He is suggesting that in those lesions, which we saw where the lumen closed up completely, it was not spasm at all. It was only a variation within the range of normal in a vessel which had an extremely thickened intima, which caused the angiographic appearance of spasm.

Dr. MacAlpin: That is one hypothesis. I do not think we can exclude by angiographic studies the possibility that there is indeed increased force of contraction of the smooth muscle against a relatively rigid vessel.

Dr. Vatner: Do you have thoughts about this other possibility?

Dr. MacAlpin: I think both possibilities exist.

Dr. Serruys: In the paper I am going to present, we have tested this hypothesis using quantitative coronary angiography and have shown that in one third of the patients we can really talk about vasomotor tone superimposed on an organic lesion. In one third of the patients at the site of the stenosis there is a kind of hypocontractile reaction and in one third of the patients there is a hypercontractility of the stenotic lesion. Indeed our impression is that for the individual it is totally unpredictable to say, which lesion is going to react like a true spasm and which lesion will react with a change in vasomotor tone superimposed on an organic lesion.

Dr. MacAlpin: Dr. Freedman from Australia presented a paper in *Circulation* last year, where he studied relatively mild stenoses of less than 50% diameter. In the patients he studied who had 'vasospastic angina,' using this kind of geometrical analysis he concluded that there had to be a shortening of the peripheral smooth muscle outside of the normal range. But these were patients who had lesser degrees of stenoses.

Dr. Bassenge: You have shown that the ergonovine effect is probably mediated by a serotonergic mechanism. So, at least in animal studies, a pretty good antagonist against ergonovine induced constriction should be methysergid, for instance or cetanserin. This would specifically block this effect which you have shown so convincingly on your angiograms. I would suggest to try that in order to see what happens in human beings under these conditions.

Dr. MacAlpin: That would be an interesting thing to do, of course. Nitroglycerin also tends to block the ergonovine action.

Dr. Chierchia: Do you think it is appropriate to extrapolate the data you have obtained with ergonovine to the normal situation in variant angina with spontaneous vasospasm? One major difference, for instance, is that if you compare spontaneously occurring spasm with vasospastic episodes induced by ergonovine in the same patient, one major feature, which is distinct in both situations is that after ergonovine administration you can see vacoconstriction of the whole coronary tree plus something superimposed at the level of the stenosis, which is not

16

neccessarily the case in spontaneously occurring episodes.

Dr. MacAlpin: Well, we have seen examples of both and I do not think that angiographically I could tell you the difference. In the patients who had spontaneous attacks of spasm, the same has occurred; that means, normal segments of the vessel go into spasm and the other coronary arteries, not involved with these spasm, constrict. There is a generalized constriction of the entire coronary artery, not just the local area. But the number of our observations is not large, so it certainly cannot be considered definitive.

Dr. Chierchia: Should the geometric theory apply to the vast majority of patients, we should expect to see other vasoconstrictors active on that lesion. If you take for instance patients with a positive response to ergonovine and you compare the response to other powerful vasoactive agents, such as angiotensin and pitressin, none of them responds, suggesting that there is something peculiar at the site of lesion, produced by ergonovine. And another observation: In the same patient with apparently the same degree of coronary lesion which may at one time respond to ergonovine, two weeks later the test may be negative. Can you comment on this as well.

Dr. MacAlpin: I agree whole heartedly with what you have said, but I have no explanation for it.

Dr. McGregor: If I could comment, and ask a question. Does that mean that you know that angiotensin has the same effect on coronary conduction vessels as does ergonovine?

Dr. Chierchia: It appears to produce diffuse vasoconstriction in some patients.

Dr. McGregor: By vasoconstriction do you mean a rise in resistance?

Dr. Chierchia: No, a reduction in diameter of the epicardial vessels.

Dr. McGregor: Then angiotensin is a good one to constrict or of epicardial vessels?

Dr. Chierchia: Yes, but it does not appear to cause coronary vessel spasm that was the meaning of my comment.

Dr. MacAlpin: I think there are a number of things that have to be considered, one of which is the effect of the vasoconstrictor on the peripheral vessels and the amount of blood-pressure rise they produce. In order to get vasoconstriction of a coronary artery there is a very close relation between the distending pressure from the inside and the constricting effect of the smooth muscle.

In animals it is extremely easy to overcome the smooth muscle effects by increasing the blood pressure sufficiently; the vessel dilates and you mask the active vasoconstriction that occurs. So with some vasoactive drugs, such as phenylephrine perhaps and angiotensin, you may cause a rise in the distending pressure to counter the vasoconstrictive effect. Ergonovine seems to have a lesser effect on the blood pressure.

Dr. Chierchia: In the experimental animal, despite increase in distending pressure and the aortic pressure by methoxamine, the coronary diameter goes down suggesting, if there is enough action on the coronary circulation, the diameter goes down inspite of an increase in distending pressure. Nevertheless, methoxamine or phenylepinephrine are not able to produce spasm in any patients in our experience.

Dr. McGregor: I do not think that you both disagree. You would not dispute that vessel tone and distending pressure are both relevant as Dr. MacAlpin said.

3. The concept of dynamic coronary stenoses

W. RAFFLENBEUL

The current understanding of the pathogenesis of myocardial ischemia is primarily based either on the concept of a high-grade 'fixed' coronary artery obstruction or a spastic vasoconstriction of an epicardial coronary artery. Both of these mechanism do not sufficiently explain the variable clinical syndromes of angina pectoris, particularly not the variation in anginal threshold experienced by many patients. Therefore, the concept of a variable vasoconstriction ('functional component') superimposed on an atherosclerotic lesion ('organic component') constitutes a plausible hypothesis connecting both pathogenic mechanisms.

The encroachment of an atherosclerotic plaque into a vessel lumen represents an additional resistance in a vessel segment which normally poses only a neglectible resistance to flow [4]. The hemodynamic consequences of this additional resistance are determined by three different factors: (1) coronary flow, (2) autoregulation on the arteriolar level and (3) the minimal residual area within the lesion.

Corresponding to the experimental data of Furuse et al. [1], Gould et al. [2], May et al. [6] and Mates et al. [5], Figure 1 demonstrates that in low- to medium-range obstructions each coronary blood flow demanded by myocardial metabolism can be delivered following reduction of autoregulatory resistance. In high-grade obstructions, however, the lesion becomes the main resistance to flow irrespective of maximal arteriolar vasodilation.

Although the application of Poiseuille's law to the human arterial system can be regarded as an oversimplification, it does serve to remind us of the major factors contributing to the pressure drop across a coronary artery stenosis. Poiseuille's relationship states that the resistance of a coronary artery stenosis is directly proportional to the length of the stenosis and the viscosity of blood and inversely proportional to the fourth power of the radius or – for a circular cross section – to the second power of the area in this stenosis:

$$\Delta P = Q \cdot \frac{8L\eta}{r_i^4} \qquad \Delta P = \bar{V} \cdot \frac{8L\eta}{r_i^2} \; ,$$

where ΔP = mean pressure gradient between two points A and B, L = length of the segment, Q = flow per unit time, $\bar{V}$ = mean velocity of fluid, r_i = inside radius

Kupper, W. (ed.), Coronary tone in ischemic heart disease. ISBN 0-89838-646-2.
© 1984, Martinus Nijhoff Publishers, Boston/The Hague/Dordrecht/Lancaster. Printed in the Netherlands.

20

and η = fluid viscosity (after Strandness [8]).

From this law an *exponential* relationship between the degree of stenosis and its resistance originates as depicted in Figure 2 for an 'idealized' obstruction in an epicardial coronary artery. The characteristics of the obstruction are given in the upper left corner: it is located in a vessel segment with a normal diameter (D_{NORM}) of 3 mm; the stenosis length is 5 mm and the flow across the stenosis should be constantly Q = 80 ml/min. The most obstructed diameter (D_{STEN}) is plotted on the lower abscissa and the calculated area stenosis on the upper abscissa. On the ordinate the resistance exerted by this obstruction is plotted as pressure gradient (ΔP) in mmHg. The ΔP was calculated according to experimental formulas [6, 8]. ΔP includes a factor for the pressure drop over the stenotic segment itself (ΔP_s), a factor for the contraction resistance (ΔP_c) at the entry of the stenosis and another factor for the pressure drop due to expansion at the stenosis-outlet (ΔP_E). The calculated diameter–resistance relationship shows a steep exponential slope starting at a diameter of about 1.6 mm, corresponding to a 65% area stenosis. In obstructions ranging from 70–90%, minute changes of the narrowest diameter result in profound changes of the stenotic resistance. For example, an increase of D_{STEN} from 1.0–1.1 mm drops the pressure gradient in this particular stenosis almost 30 mmHg.

From this relationship it is readily recognizable that vasoconstriction superimposed on a pre-existing atherosclerotic lesion easily transfers a medium-grade stenosis into a high-grade flow limiting obstruction. To produce such aggravation

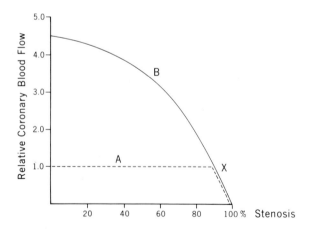

Figure 1. Relationship between relative coronary blood flow (ordinate) – 1.0 is the resting flow – and the degree of a coronary artery stenosis (abscissa). Curve A represents the resting flow maintained constant due to successive reduction of arteriolar resistance. Curve B illustrates maximal coronary blood flow after maximal arteriolar vasodilation (coronary reserve). At point X basal flow cannot longer be supplied despite maximal arteriolar vasodilation, i.e. the point of 'critical' stenosis which degree of severity may shift with coronary blood flow demanded by myocardial metabolism.

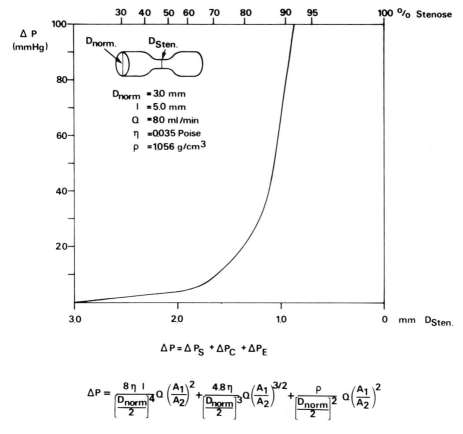

$$\Delta P = \Delta P_S + \Delta P_C + \Delta P_E$$

$$\Delta P = \frac{8\eta\, l}{\left[\frac{D_{norm}}{2}\right]^4}Q\left(\frac{A_1}{A_2}\right)^2 + \frac{4.8\eta}{\left[\frac{D_{norm}}{2}\right]^3}Q\left(\frac{A_1}{A_2}\right)^{3/2} + \frac{\rho}{\left[\frac{D_{norm}}{2}\right]^2}Q\left(\frac{A_1}{A_2}\right)^2$$

Figure 2. Schematic relationship between the severity of a coronary stenosis (abscissa) and the pressure gradient ΔP across this stenosis (ordinate) under constant coronary flow conditions. See text for details.

of stenosis severity the rhythmic changes of coronary artery diameters already reported by Gensini 1971 are sufficient. Furthermore, recent research has demonstrated that an atherogenic lipid invironment increases coronary vessel wall sensitivity to vasoconstrictor stimuli [3]. In addition, the development of an atherosclerotic plaque in vascular areas with angiographically proven spasm may illustrate the close relationship between vasoconstriction, intimal lesion and the triggering of the atherosclerotic process [7].

Figure 3 illustrates an example of a vasoconstriction superimposed on a medium range coronary artery stenosis. The most obstructed diameter (D_{STEN}) of 1.40 mm – corresponding to a 82% area stenosis – dilated to 1.96 mm, i.e. about 40% after sublingual application of 0.8 mg nitroglycerin plus 20 mg nifedipine. In our experience increased vascular smooth muscle tone superimposed on a coronary stenosis seems to be a relatively common mechanism aggravating stenosis

22

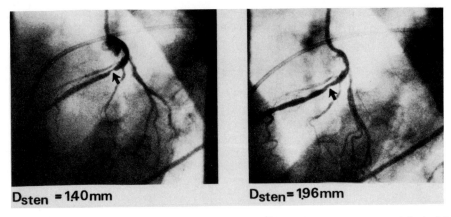

$D_{sten} = 1.40\,mm$ $D_{sten} = 1.96\,mm$

Figure 3. Angiographic example of a vasoconstriction superimposed on a coronary stenosis in the left anterior descending coronary artery. After the combined sublingual application of 0.8 mg of nitroglycerin plus 20 mg of nifedipine the most obstructed diameter within the stenosis (D_{STEN}) dilated from 1.40 mm to 1.96 mm, i.e. about 40%.

severity, as depicted in Figure 4. The combined sublingual application of 0.8 mg nitroglycerin plus 20 mg nifedipine on 50 consecutive patients with coronary obstructions with variable severity resulted in a considerable increase of D_{STEN} in 31 out of the 50 obstructions with an average dilatation of +49%. Only in 19 stenoses no vasodilatory effect could be demonstrated.

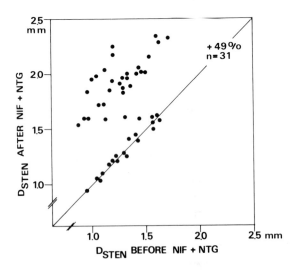

Figure 4. Combined effect of 20 mg nifedipine plus 0.8 mg of nitroglycerin s.l. on the most obstructed diameter (D_{STEN}) of 50 coronary artery stenoses with variable severity D_{STEN} increased significantly in 31 obstructions with an average diameter increase of +49%.

Clinically this concept of 'dynamic' changes in the degree of coronary artery stenosis might be relevant in patients with a variable threshold of angina pectoris. It seems conceivable that in these patients the symptoms vary according to two independent factors: (1) the severity of the atherosclerotic lesion and (2) the extend of the superimposed vasoconstriction due to increased tone of vascular smooth muscle. Particularly because of the relatively quick changes in vascular tone the onset of angina pectoris during exertion or even at rest might vary in these patients afflicted with coronary artery disease.

References

1. Furuse A, Klopp EH, Brawley RK, Gott VL: Hemodynamics of aorto-to-coronary artery bypass. Ann Thorac Surg 14:282, 1972.
2. Gould KL, Lipscomb K, Calvert D: Compensatory changes of the distal coronary vascular bed during progressive coronary restriction. Circulation 51:1085, 1975.
3. Henry PD, Yokoyama M: Inappropriate coronary vasomotion: search for a local fault. In: Rafflenbeul W, Lichtlen P, Balcon R (eds) Unstable Angina Pectoris. Georg Thieme Verlag, Stuttgart, 1981.
4. Klocke FJ: Coronary blood flow in man. Prog Cardiovasc Dis 19:117, 1976.
5. Mates RE, Gupta RL, Bell AC, Klocke FJ: Fluid dynamics of coronary artery stenosis. Circ Res 42: 152, 1978.
6. May AG, DeWeese JA, Robb CG: Hemodynamic effects of arterial stenosis. Surgery 53:513, 1963.
7. Russell R: Atherosclerosis: a problem of the biology of arterial wall cells and their interactions with blood components. Atherosclerosis 1(5):2093, 1981.
8. Strandness DE (1977): Flow dynamics in circulatory pathophysiology. In: Hwang NHC, Norman NA (eds) Cardiovascular Flow Dynamics and Measurements. University Park Press, Baltimore, pp 307–324.

Discussion

Dr. McGregor: I suppose you would agree that there can be major changes in the reactivity of the vessels such as the increased ability of ergonovine to produce spasm in the immediate postinfarction period.

Dr. Rafflenbeul: These were all patients with chronic stable angina and the response should be the same in the patients we were talking about.

Dr. MacAlpin: That is very nice, but almost too good to be true. Have you looked at patients with a clinical picture consistent with vasospastic angina to see whether you could then with the use of this type of analysis from the form of the stenosis predict which patient might be susceptible to vasospastic angina and which might not?

Dr. Rafflenbeul: We tried to do this – to separate the patients concerning to their morphology – but that did not work.

4. Contribution of dynamic vascular wall thickening to luminal narrowing during coronary arterial vasomotion

P.W. SERRUYS, J.M. LABLANCHE, J.W. DECKERS,
J.H.C. REIBER, M.E. BERTRAND & P.G. HUGENHOLTZ

Introduction

When trying to establish what constitutes a physiologically significant obstruction to blood flow in the human coronary system of patients with exertional angina, we implicitly assume that the pathogenesis of exertional angina pectoris is based primarily on the concept of a 'fixed' stenosis that causes angina when flow requirements of the myocardium exceed the flow capacity of the diseased vessel.

Recently, the hypothesis has been developed that increased coronary arterial vasomotor tone superimposed on a pre-existing obstruction in a coronary artery is an important pathophysiologic mechanism responsible for causing angina pectoris not only at rest but also during exercise [1, 2]. On the other hand, it has been clearly established that the arteries of patients with spontaneous spasm or inappropriate vasomotor tone are hypersensitive to ergonovine at the sites of atherosclerotic lesions [3–10].

MacAlpin [11] recently proposed that this hypersensitivity was in fact due to the amplification of normal vasoconstriction at sites of atheromatous luminal encroachments, the degree of vasoconstriction being related to the severity of encroachment (geometric theory).

We undertook the present study to determine whether this geometric theory could explain the hypersensitivity of arteries in patients with vasospastic angina. Therefore, we tried to assess the amount of coronary tone present in 18 patients who were known to have complaints of exertional and resting angina by measuring the maximal changes in coronary arterial diameter induced by a provocative test (methergin) followed by an intracoronary injection of isosorbide dinitrate.

Using elementary geometric principles, we calculated and reconstructed the changes that might occur at the stenotic sites as the result of 'normal' vasomotion of the non-stenotic segment adjacent to the obstructive lesion.

Kupper, W. (ed.), Coronary tone in ischemic heart disease. ISBN 0-89838-646-2.
© *1984, Martinus Nijhoff Publishers, Boston/The Hague/Dordrecht/Lancaster. Printed in the Netherlands.*

Methods

Patient selection and vasomotor tone testing

In a highly selected group of 18 patients, who were known to have complaints of exertional and resting angina, we tried to explore the entire spectrum of coronary vasomotor tone by measuring the maximal changes in coronary arterial diameter, induced by a provocative test (bolus i.v. of 0.4 mg methylergobasine (methergin)) followed by an intracoronary injection of 3 mg isosorbide dinitrate (Risordan). A total of 20 stenotic coronary segments was selected for quantitative angiographic analysis. Before the pharmacological intervention, a base-line coronary angiogram (control) was performed. Five minutes later, 0.4 mg of methergin was injected intravenously.

A second arteriogram was obtained 5 min after the intravenous injection of methergin, or as soon as the patient developed chest pain or/and ST-T changes on his electrocardiogram.

The third coronary angiogram was recorded two minutes after an intracoronary injection of isosorbide dinitrate (3 mg Risordan).

The X-ray system was maintained in exactly the same position during the sequential angiographic studies in a particular patient, i.e. no differences in projection occurred.

Quantitative angiographic analysis system

In the present study, for each individual patient arterial dimensions were measured at specific distances from identifiable branch points in diastolic frames before and after methergin and isosorbide dinitrate administration.

The quantitative analysis of selected coronary segments was carried out with the help of a computer-based coronary angiography analysis system (CAAS); which has been described extensively elsewhere [12–14].

To analyze a selected 35-mm cineframe, the film is placed on a specially constructed cine-video converter. This converter consists of a standard 35-mm Vanguard cinefilm transport mechanism, a drum with six different lens systems allowing the selection of the desired optical magnification and a high resolution video camera mounted on a motordriven x–y stage [12]. By means of this cine-video converter any portion of the 35-mm cineframe can be selected with the appropriate magnification factor. The cinefilm transport, the selection of the optical magnification as well as the x–y positioning of the video camera are all operated through a PDP 11/44 host computer. The magnified portion of the cineframe is displayed on a video monitor; in practice, an optical magnification factor of two is used for the coronary segments. Regions of interest in the image can be digitized and stored into computer memory for subsequent processing. Graphics and the computer detected contours of a coronary arterial segment can be superimposed in the video image displayed on the monitor. Operator interaction is possible with a writing table.

The computerized analysis of a selected coronary segment requires the manual definition of a number of center positions within the segment by means of a writing table. A smooth continuous curve, the centerline, is subsequently generated through these center positions. This centerline determines the regions of interest of size 96×96 pixels, encompassing the arterial segments to be digitized. Contour positions are detected along scanlines perpendicular to the local centerline directions on the basis of a minimum cost contour detection algorithm [14]. The cost of a pixel is defined as the inverse of the weighted sum of the first- and second-derivative value of the brightness information. If the user does not agree with part of the detected contours, these positions may be corrected interactively. On the basis of the detected contour positions a new centerline is computed and the contour detection procedure is repeated. This interactive approach has been implemented to minimize the influence of the user definition of the center points on the detected contours. Finally, a smoothing procedure is applied to each of the contours. As a next step, all the contour positions are corrected for pincushion distortion introduced by the image intensifier. For each pixel in the image a correction vector was previously assessed from a digitized image of a cm-grid and stored in memory.

Calibration of the diameter data is achieved by using the intra-cardiac catheter as a scaling device. To this end, the contours of part of the projected catheter are detected automatically in a way similar as described above for the arterial segment; in addition, a priori information is included in the iterative edge detection procedure based on the fact that the selected part of the catheter is the projection of a cylindrical structure. The optical magnification factor for the catheter is usually chosen as $2\sqrt{2}$. A mean diameter value is determined in pixels, so that the calibration factor can be computed from the known size of the catheter.

From the final contours, the diameter (D)-function is determined by computing the shortest distances between the left and right contour positions (curves in Figures 1A–C). As a next step the computer algorithm determines the position of the obstruction by searching for the minimal diameter value in the diameter function. This position can be changed interactively by the user if more than one focal obstruction is to be processed within the analyzed arterial segment. The extent of the selected obstruction is determined from the diameter function on the basis of curvature analysis and expressed in mm. The detected boundaries of the obstruction are indicated in the D-function with two dotted lines. For the purpose of determining the percentage diameter reduction of an obstruction the reference diameter is computed as the average of 11 diameter values in a symmetric region with center at a user-defined reference position.

For parts of the analyzed segments proximal and/or distal of the obstructions,

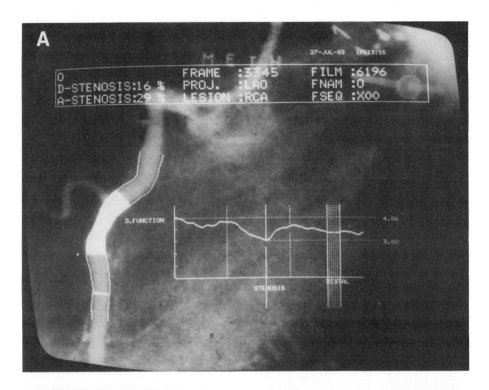

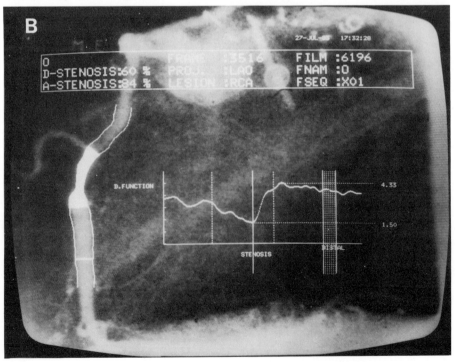

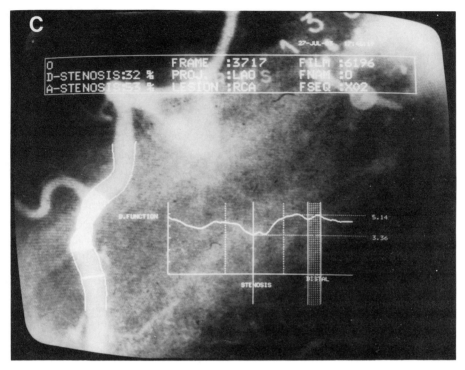

Figure 1. Computer output of an analyzed lesion in the right coronary artery at different states of vasomotion: (A) control state, (B) after intravenous methergin, (C) after intracoronary isosorbide dinitrate.

which show no abnormalities in sizes, mean proximal and/or distal diameters can be computed, respectively. To this end the user indicates the two boundary positions of such parts with the writing tablet and the mean diameter values are computed.

The accuracy of the quantification method has been validated with perspex models of coronary arteries with circular cross-sections. The diameter reduction percentages as well as absolute obstruction dimensions of the models were measured with the described procedure for various settings of the X-ray system and with different concentrations of the contrast agent. The average deviation from the true values for the percentages diameter stenosis equaled 2.00% ± 2.32% (mean ± SD) and for the absolute minimal obstruction diameter −0.03 ± 0.10 mm (mean ± SD) [14].

Geometric considerations: dynamic vascular wall thickening

Quantitation of vasomotion observed by angiography is limited to comparing the luminal diameter in two or more states of vasomotion. Because we cannot see the arterial wall itself, we do not always appreciate the changes occurring in it that produce the variations in luminal dimensions, we call 'vasomotion' [11, 15, 16].

The elementary geometric principle used to predict the narrowing expected at a lesion site, given the severity of the lesion and the degree of vasoconstriction of the adjacent normal segment, is shown in Figures 2, 3 and 4.

Let us assume a coronary artery that is circular in cross section when distended by a normal blood pressure and has an outer diameter $2R_o$ (e.g. 2.4 mm) including the media but excluding the adventitia (Figure 2). Furthermore, there is a coronary obstruction in the segment under consideration with a minimal (luminal) obstruction diameter $2r_i$ (1.4 mm); the luminal reference diameter in the normal prestenotic segment equals $2R_i$ (2.0 mm).

Figure 3 shows the cross sections at the reference position and at the site of the obstruction with the definitions of the different radii. The area A_R of the arterial wall at the reference cross section equals $A_R = (R_o^2 - R_i^2)$ and the area A_s at the obstruction $A_s = (R_o^2 - r_i^2)$. These diameter and area values define the control situation.

A new situation is created as vasoconstriction occurs (Figures 2 and 4). For practical purposes, the material of the arterial wall is plastic but not incompressible. If we assume that there is no change in the length of the artery as the result of

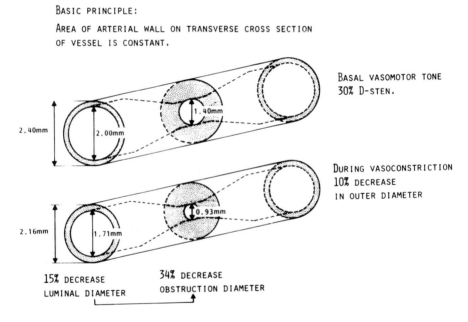

BASIC PRINCIPLE:
AREA OF ARTERIAL WALL ON TRANSVERSE CROSS SECTION
OF VESSEL IS CONSTANT.

BASAL VASOMOTOR TONE
30% D-STEN.

2.40mm   2.00mm   1.40mm

DURING VASOCONSTRICTION
10% DECREASE
IN OUTER DIAMETER

2.16mm   1.71mm   0.93mm

15% DECREASE
LUMINAL DIAMETER

34% DECREASE
OBSTRUCTION DIAMETER

Figure 2. Contribution of dynamic vascular wall thickening to luminal narrowing during coronary arterial constriction.

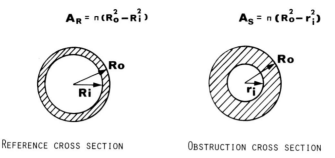

$$A_R = \pi(R_o^2 - R_i^2)$$

$$A_s = \pi(R_o^2 - r_i^2)$$

Figure 3. A hypothetical coronary artery with circular cross sections (A_R and A_s) at a prestenotic reference position and at the site of a coronary obstruction, respectively.

changes in its diameter, and no extrusion of tissue from the constricted area into non-constricted, adjacent parts of the artery, then at any point of the artery the area of the arterial wall on a transverse cross section of the vessel will be constant regardless of the state of its contraction or dilation. If we denote the new outer diameter Roc, the luminal obstruction diameter ric and the reference diameter Ric in the state of vasoconstriction, then the following equations hold:

$$A_r = (Roc^2 - Ric^2) = (Ro^2 - Ri^2) \tag{1}$$
$$\text{or} \quad Ro^2 - Roc^2 = Ri^2 - Ric^2 \tag{2}$$

$$\text{and} \quad A_s = (Roc^2 - ric^2) = (Ro^2 - ri^2) \tag{3}$$
$$\text{or} \quad Ro^2 - Roc^2 = ri^2 - ric^2 \tag{4}$$

Then (2) and (4) yield:
$$ric^2 = ri^2 - Ri^2 + Ric^2 \tag{5}$$

Thus if we know the reference diameter in the control state (Ri) and after vasoconstriction (Ric) and the obstruction diameter ri in the control state, then we can predict the minimal obstruction diameter ric after vasoconstriction from equation (5).

It should be clear, that the equations (1)–(5) are equally valid for vasoconstriction and vasodilation situations.

At the top of Figure 2 we see a coronary stenotic lesion with a 30% diameter stenosis in the basal condition.

Now let us assume that a 10% decrease in the outer diameter occurs as a result of vasoconstriction, that is the outer diameter becomes 2.16 mm (bottom drawing of Figure 2). Under the assumption of a constant transverse cross section it can be derived from the simple geometric principles given above that a 15% decrease occurs in the luminal diameter of the prestenotic segment.

At the stenotic site, because of the modest mural thickening due to disease, the luminal diameter decreases in greater proportion; in the present case a 34% decrease in obstruction diameter can be predicted from equation (5).

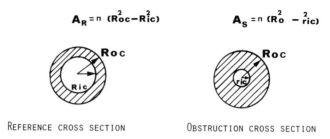

$$A_R = \pi \, (R_{oc}^2 - R_{ic}^2) \qquad\qquad A_S = \pi \, (R_o^2 - r_{ic}^2)$$

REFERENCE CROSS SECTION   OBSTRUCTION CROSS SECTION

Figure 4. Cross sections of Figure 3 after vasoconstriction.

Results (Table 1)

The effects of methergin i.v. and isosorbide dinitrate i.c. on the mean proximal diameter and on the minimal obstruction diameter are shown in Figure 5. The differences in value that may be seen in Table 1 between the reference diameter and mean proximal diameter stem from the fact, that the reference diameter is computed over only 11 pixel positions, which corresponds to a width of approximately 1 mm whereas the mean proximal diameter is usually computed over a much larger length, e.g. over 100–200 pixel positions or approximately 10–20 mm wide.

During the provocative test the mean proximal diameter decreases significantly ($p<0.005$) by 11%, with respect to the basal condition, from 3.7 to 3.3 mm, whereas the minimal obstruction diameter is reduced by more than 50% from 2.2 to 1.0 mm ($p<10^{-7}$). The intracoronary injection of isosorbide dinitrate provokes a very significant vasodilation of the obstructive lesion from 1.0 mm to 2.7 mm ($p<10^{-8}$), as well as a significant increase in mean proximal diameter from 3.3 mm to 4.2 mm ($p<10^{-6}$).

The individual changes in minimal obstruction diameter are given in Figure 6.

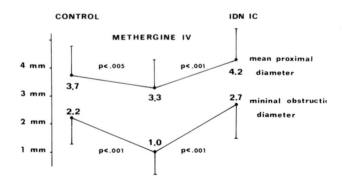

Figure 5. Effects of methergin® intravenous (IV) and of isosorbide intracoronary (IC) on the mean proximal diameter and on the minimal obstruction diameter; n = 20.

After methergin six (marked with arrows in Figure 6) of the twenty analysed stenotic lesions became transiently occluded, whereas isosorbide dinitrate i.c. increased the luminal diameters of all the obstructive lesions, which were vasoconstricted during the provocative test.

In terms of percentage diameter stenosis, the severity of the obstructive lesions increased on the average from 41% to 70% (p<0.0001) during the provocative test and returned to an average value of 36% after the intracoronary injection of isosorbide dinitrate (Figure 7).

Then, using the elementary geometric principles described above in the methods, we calculated and reconstructed the changes that might occur at the stenotic sites as the results of vasomotion acting on the entire coronary segment.

In Figure 8, the decrease of luminal diameter of a normal prestenotic segment is plotted against the expected decrease in luminal diameter of the stenotic segment for a stenosis with a 20% diameter reduction. For this example a 20% decrease in luminal diameter of the normal segment causes a 33% decrease in diameter of the stenotic segment.

When applying this theoretical relationship to the different states of vasomotion measured in our group of 18 patients, we found that the behavior of the stenotic lesions during vasoconstriction deviated considerably from this theoretical relationship, some stenotic lesions being hypercontractile, and some others being hypocontractile (Figure 9).

As a matter of fact, during vasoconstriction only four stenotic lesions did react as predicted by the theory and we can conclude that their decrease in luminal diameter at the stenotic sites was simply the result of an increase in vasomotor tone superimposed on an organically narrowed vessel.

Six stenotic lesions were hypocontractile and the vessel wall at the site of the

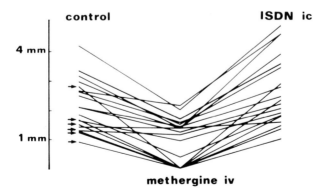

Figure 6. Individual changes in minimal obstruction diameter after methergin® iv and isosorbide dinitrate ic. Six (marked with arrows) of the 20 analyzed stenotic lesions are transiently occluded during the provocative test.

Table 1. Results from quantitative analysis of coronary arteries in different states of vasomotion.

Name			Artery	Reference diameter (mm)	Obstruction diameter (mm)	User-defined % D-sten	Mean proximal diameter (mm)	Mean distal diameter (mm)
no	1 VA	1[a]	RCA	4.93	4.20	14.9	4.89	4.75
		2	RCA	5.39	2.79	28.3	5.24	4.33
		3	RCA	6.03	4.88	19.0	5.76	5.19
no	2 Gh	1	LAD	2.80	0.90	68.0	2.70	3.70
		2	LAD		totally occluded		2.10	
		3	LAD	3.01	1.76	41.4	2.99	3.48
no	3 O1	1	RCA	4.48	3.34	25.4	4.1	3.8
		2	RCA	3.22	1.68	47.8	3.14	4.2 1
		3	RCA	4.15	3.57	14.0	4.36	4.99
	O1	1	RCA	4.04	3.34	17.3	4.1	3.8
		2	RCA	4.14	1.68	59.4	3.14	4.21
		3	RCA	5.02	3.57	28.8	4.36	4.99
no	4 Be	1	RCA	5.96	2.79	53.2	5.82	4.46
		2	RCA		totally occluded		4.98	
		3	RCA	6.36	2.88	54.7	6.52	5.97
no	5 Cr	1	RCA	5.34	3.16	40.9	5.21	
		2	RCA	5.11	1.37	73.1	4.85	
		3	RCA	5.29	3.90	26.3	5.26	
no	6 Flc	1	RCA	3.73	1.63	56.3	3.72	
		2	RCA	3.63	0.94	74.1	3.55	
		3	RCA	4.01	1.88	53.1	4.09	
	Flc	1	RCA	3.73	2.09	43.8	3.72	
		2	RCA	3.52	1.42	59.6	3.55	
		3	RCA	3.98	2.44	38.6	4.09	
no	7 Duf	1	RCA	3.21	2.62	18.6	3.65	3.15
		2	RCA	2.21	1.56	29.5	3.24	2.22
		3	RCA	3.00	2.77	7.7	3.83	2.97
no	8 Flm	1	RCA	4.75	2.48	47.7	4.80	4.25
		2	RCA	4.02	1.36	66.2	4.00	2.54
		3	RCA	5.30	4.59	13.3	5.29	4.21
no	9 Dup	1	LCX	5.88	2.65	54.9	6.11	3.69
		2	LCX	4.94	2.14	56.7	4.73	3.62
		3	LCX	7.01	4.59	34.6	7.02	5.11
no 10	Ti	1	LAD	2.38	1.22	48.7	2.36	2.62
		2	LAD		totally occluded		2.16	
		3	LAD	3.39	1.44	57.6	3.18	2.69
no 11	No	1	RCA	3.16	1.83	42.0		3.16
		2	RCA	2.89	0.38	86.7		2.76
		3	RCA	3.31	1.79	45.9		3.16
no 12	De	1	RCA	3.11	1.49	52.0	3.04	3.54
		2	RCA		totally occluded		2.38	
		3	RCA	3.94	0.99	74.9	3.88	3.77

Table 1. (continued).

Name		Artery	Reference diameter (mm)	Obstruction diameter (mm)	User-defined % D-sten	Mean proximal diameter (mm)	Mean distal diameter (mm)
no 13 Dum	1	LAD	3.23	1.29	60.1	3.08	
	2	LAD	2.67	1.14	57.3	2.70	
	3	LAD	3.97	2.03	49.0	3.96	
no 14 Paz	1	LAD	2.43	1.27	47.6		2.41
	2	LAD		totally occluded		2.64	
	3	LAD	3.58	2.32	35.4	2.60	3.22
no 15 Pat	1	LAD	2.85	2.09	26.8		2.70
	2	LAD	2.31	1.23	46.6		2.05
	3	LAD	2.82	2.19	22.2		2.71
no 16 Me	1	RCA	3.75	2.96	21.0	2.83	
	2	RCA	4.24	1.50	64.6	3.94	2.70
	3	RCA	3.60	3.44	4.5	3.55	3.69
no 17 Gr	1	LAD	3.24	1.65	49.0	3.06	3.36
	2	LAD		totally occluded		2.70	
	3	LAD	3.38	1.33	60.8	3.50	3.0
no 18 Jo	1	RCA	2.94	1.41	51.9		2.98
	2	RCA	1.98	1.37	30.7		1.94
	3	RCA	2.90	1.56	46.3	2.88	3.39

[a] 1 = control, 2 = methergin, 3 = isosorbide dinitrate.
Abbreviations: RCA (right coronary artery); LAD (left anterior descending artery); LCX (left circumflex artery).

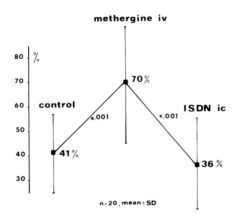

Figure 7. Changes in percentage diameter stenosis during the provocative test and after the intracoronary injection of isosorbide dinitrate.

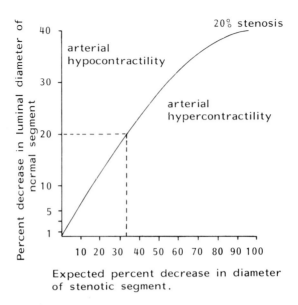

Figure 8. The percent decrease in luminal diameter of a normal prestenotic segment is plotted against the expected decrease in luminal diameter of the stenotic segment for a stenosis with a 20% diameter reduction.

lesion actually constricted less than suggested by the theoretical model. In five cases we even predicted a total occlusion which was not observed.

As for the 12 remaining lesions, they all showed arterial hypercontractility and four of them, unexpectedly, became totally occluded during vasoconstriction.

Discussion

The present study demonstrates, in patients with exertional and resting angina, the unpredictability of diameter changes at stenotic sites when a vasoconstrictor agent like methergin is given. Our results are not in agreement with MacAlpin's geometric theory, which postulates that dynamic narrowing of stenotic lesions is a direct and predictable consequence of the luminal encroachment by atheroma and the resulting increase in wall area on a transverse cross section at this point. In other words, according to MacAlpin, a modest mural thickening due to disease may act as a 'lever' in translating physiologic degrees of medial smooth muscle shortening into critical luminal obstruction.

Only four out of 22 stenotic lesions in our group of patients reacted as prognosticated by this theory. Angiographic observations by Freedman et al. [10] could neither be explained by MacAlpin's theoretical consideration. They compared the vasoconstrictor effect of ergonovine in 11 patients with variant angina and in 21 patients with atypical chest pain. The dynamic response of the stenotic lesions in patients with variant angina – in contrast to the reaction in the patients with atypical complaints – was always more pronounced than predicted by the geometric theory, although atheromateous lesions in both groups of patients were similar. Their results suggest an increased sensitivity of the obstructive lesion to ergonovine in patients with variant angina. Although the reason for hypersensitivity to ergonovine at sites of atheroma is unknown, Henry and Yokoyama [17] recently suggested that the supersensitivity of atherosclerotic arteries to ergonovine in rabbits with diet induced atherosclerosis was mediated by a serotonergic mechanism, which could not be inhibited by alpha adrenergic blockers [17]. Furthermore, it has been reported that H-1 receptor stimulation by histamine also induced coronary artery spasm in some patients [18], suggesting a causal cellular mechanism beyond the level of interaction between a single agonist and its membrane receptor.

Observations in our study, in a homogeneous group of patients, demonstrate, after ergonovine, an arterial hypercontractility in 12 of the 22 stenotic lesions,

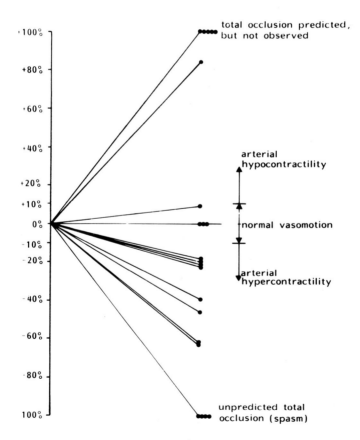

Figure 9. Percentage deviation of the obstruction diameters from predicted values after methergin.

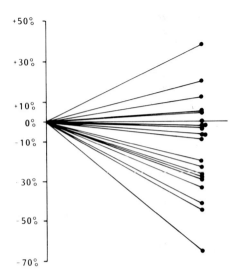

Figure 10. Percentage deviation of the obstruction diameters form predicted values after isosorbide dinitrate i.c.

whereas an unexplained hypocontractility was found at six other sites.

Elucidation of this latter phenomenon, could be either a decreased pliability of the coronary artery at the site of an atherosclerotic plaque [11], or the destruction of smooth muscle by the atherosclerotic process [10]. Technical shortcomings, i.e. the use of a single angiographic view, could also underestimate the contraction of the flexible part of an eccentric stenosis.

In contrast to the unpredictable coronary vasoconstriction after ergonovine, vasodilatation by intracoronary isosorbide dinitrate occurred in all patients, and at all stenotic sites. Vasodilatation in about half of the segments could be accurately predicted by MacAlpin's theory. We conclude from our data that the extent of vasoconstriction due to ergonovine in patients with exertional and resting angina is unpredictable and not adequately explained by geometric principles. Vasodilatation at stenotic sites by isosorbide dinitrate, however, is a more predictable event, which can to a larger extent be accounted for by MacAlpin's geometric theory.

References

1. Serruys PW, Steward R, Booman F, Michels R, Reiber JHC, Hugenholtz PG: Can unstable angina pectoris be due to increased coronary vasomotor tone? Eur Heart J 1(suppl B):71, 1980.
2. Epstein SE, Talbot TL: Dynamic coronary tone in precipitation, exacerbation and relief of angina pectoris. Am J Cardiol 48:797, 1981.
3. Maseri A, Severi S, DeNes M, L'Abbate A, Chierchia S, Marzilli M, Ballestra AM, Parodi O,

Biagine A, Distante A: 'Variant' angina: one aspect of a continuous spectrum of vasospastic myocardial ischaemia. Am J Cardiol 42:1019, 1978.

4. MacAlpin RN: Relation of coronary arterial spasm to sites of organic stenosis. Am J Cardiol 46:143, 1980.

5. Heupler FA, Proudfit WL, Razavi M, Shirey EK, Greenstreet R, Sheldon WC: Ergonovine maleate provocative test for coronary arterial spasm. Am J Cardiol 41:631, 1978.

6. Schroeder JS, Bolen JL, Quint RA, Clark DA, Hayden WG, Higgins CB, Wexler L. Provocation of coronary spasm with ergonovine maleate. Am J Cardiol 40:487, 1977.

7. Waters DD, Theroux P, Szlachcic J, Dauwe F, Crittin J, Bonan R, Mizgala HF: Ergonovine testing in a coronary care unit. Am J Cardiol 46:922, 1980.

8. Curry RC, Pepine CJ, Sabom MB, Feldman RL, Christie LG, Conti CR: Effects of ergonovine in patients with and without coronary artery disease. Circulation 56:803, 1977.

9. Freedman SB, Dunn RF, Bernstein L, Richmond DR, O'Neill G, Kelly DT: Coronary artery spasm: use of ergonovine in diagnosis. Aust NZ J Med 10:6, 1980.

10. Freedman B, Richmond DR, Kelly DT: Pathophysiology of coronary artery spasm. Circulation 66:705, 1982.

11. MacAlpin RN: Contribution of dynamic vascular wall thickening to luminal narrowing during coronary arterial constriction. Circulation 61:296, 1980.

12. Reiber JHC, Gerbrands JJ, Kooijman CJ, et al: Quantitative coronary angiography with automated contour detection and densitometry; technical aspects. In: Just H, Heintzen PH (eds) Angiocardiography, Current Status and Future Developments. Springer-Verlag, Heidelberg, 1983.

13. Reiber JHC, Gerbrands JJ, Booman F, et al: Objective characterization of coronary obstructions from monoplane cineangiograms and three-dimensional reconstruction of an arterial segment from orthogonal views. In: Schwartz MD (ed) Application of Computers in Medicine. IEEE Cat No Th 0095-0, 1982, pp 93–100.

14. Kooijman CJ, Reiber JHC, Gerbrands JJ, et al: Computer-aided quantitation of the severity of coronary obstructions from single view cineangiograms. International Symposium on medical imaging and image interpretation. IEEE Cat No 82CH1804-4, 1982, pp 59–64.

15. Folkow B, Grimby G, Thulesius O: Adaptive structural changes of the vascular walls in hypertension and their relation to the control of the peripheral resistance. Acta Physiol Scand 44:255, 1958.

16. Conway J: Vascular reactivity in experimental hypertension measured after hexamethonium. Circulation 17:807, 1958.

17. Henry PD, Yokoyama M: Supersensitivity of atherosclerotic rabbit aorta to ergonovine: mediation by a serotonergic mechanism. J Clin Invest 66:306, 1980.

18. Ginsburg R, Bristow MR, Kantrowwitz N, et al: Histamine provocation of clinical coronary artery spasm: implications concerning pathogenesis of variant angina pectoris. Am Heart J 102(5):819–82, 1981.

Discussion

Dr. Kupper: During your ergonovine-intervention you sometimes found a considerable reduction in obstruction diameter in patients with an unpredicted spasm. I may have missed it, but how many of these patients developed angina or ST-segment changes during the intervention?

Dr. Serruys: Six patients developed ST-elevation (these were the six patients with the total occlusion of the vessel) and in four of the patients there was ST-depression during the test.

Dr. McGregor: Your conclusion is that MacAlpin's hypothesis is a contributor only in a minority of cases of apparent occlusion. Did you, by any chance, find a difference between eccentric and concentric lesions, because your technique must be able to display that very well.

Dr. Serruys: That is right, but at that time we were working only in one projection, using the technique of the automatic contour detection, but, as you can see, we are able to measure the intravascular density of the contrast material and then we are independent of shape of the lesion. I am still working on it and extending the study, looking at the cross sectional area in absolute terms during this kind of test. The preliminary results show basically the same kind of information. That means that in one third of the patients, we can talk about vasomotor tone superimposed on the lesion, but there are also lesions, which are hypoc-ontractile and I would say, they are certainly a little more concentric than the other lesions and on the other side the lesion showing after the intervention a total occlusion has certainly the tendency to be more excentric.

Dr. Bleifeld: What about the accuracy of your system. I ask that because if you make a magnification you also increase the error of your measurements.

Dr. Serruys: We have tested the system in perspex models starting under static and dynamic flow conditions and in collaboration with Dr. Rafflenbeul we compared post-mortem lesions with in vivo coronary angiograms and it was shown that the resolution of the system is excellent.

Dr. Dickenson: I just wonder whether there is another factor that comes in. I remember that before electromagnetic flow meters were used, one of the ways to measure flow was to make a constriction on a tube and then measure the pressure difference between pre- and poststenotic area. The faster the flow, the lower the pressure was inside the stenotic region. It seems paradox, but you have a greater kinetic energy in the fluid flowing through the stenosis, so the distending pressure in the stenosis is in fact less, the faster the flow. And I wonder if that is not possibly a contributor.

I was much struck of the combined impact of the first three papers. May be if you start up with a normal elastic coronary artery and you get a stenotic plaque than there might be a point, from which you will get a vicious circle, as the diameter gets less and less and the intravascular flow speeds up, especially if there is a low pressure distally. The distending pressure will get less and less and so you will have a tendency for the stenosis to close up. I mean, is this completely naive?

Dr. Serruys: I think this is not naive, there are a lot of papers from Santamoore and Walinsky on collapsing stenotic lesions, induced by a reduction in what they call the distending pressure.

If I remember well, the main criticism of Gould on this hypothesis was that in a clinical situation especially in the human being, when you are doing intracoronary injection of a vasodilatory drug, then you are not only dilating the distal part of the coronary artery, which was done in the study by Walinsky and Santamoore, but you also dilate the pre-, the stenotic, and the post-stenotic segment.

On the other hand, we have measured during PTCA the gradient across the lesion. When we injected intracoronary nifedipine distal to the stenotic lesion, we had a vasodilation only of the distal part of the vessel. And we were unable to demonstrate this collapse of the stenosis in human beings.

Dr. Bassenge: The law of Lambert-Beer applies only to very diluted solutions, which is certainly not the case in blood mixed with contrast medium. Therefore, I wonder about the accuracy of your measurements?

Dr. Serruys: That is a very good question. It is right that we have to calibrate the system and the entire optical chain before the study, using different grey scales and different qualities of the cine film first. The second aspect of the problem is that the distribution of the contrast material within the stenosis could be different in the pre- and post-stenotic region. So we tested the density of the contrast medium at the stenotic site in the vessel under various conditions including pulsatile blood flow and it did not seem to be a major problem. The major problem could be the distance between the tip of the catheter and the lesion, because you really need good mixing of the blood and contrast material before reaching the lesion, if you want to have an accurate measurement. So possibly in very proximal lesions of the LAD, this could be a problem.

5. Alteration in coronary vasomotor tone by alpha-stimulation

E. BASSENGE & J. HOLTZ

1. Introduction

The concept of the dynamic coronary artery stenosis in its extreme form, the coronary spasm, has substantially extended our understanding of coronary heart disease [1–6]. The revitalization of this old concept has been triggered by Prinzmetal's careful observations of patients with variant forms of angina pectoris [7]. Besides the significant impact for diagnosis and therapy of angina this concept concomitantly restimulated interest in the physiologic role of constrictive mechanisms in the coronary bed, especially of the sympathetic coronary innervation. As summarized recently [8], anecdotal observations in patients indicate that α-adrenoceptor mediated coronary constriction might be an attractive hypothesis for one of several possible pathophysiological mechanisms of coronary spasms, for which conclusive evidence is lacking. One reason for this uncertainty concerning the pathophysiologic relevance of α-adrenoceptor mediated corornary constriction results from the difficulties in assessing its role under physiologic conditions. There is general agreement that, in studies under β-blockade, a coronary constriction can be elicited by activation of coronary α-adrenoceptors in most mammals including man and that these α-adrenoceptors are functionally innervated (i.e. that they can be activated by norepinephrine released from nerve endings (for reviews see [9]). However, the significance of these α-adrenoceptors relative to the role of coronary vascular β-adrenoceptors and to metabolic coronary regulation is highly controversial.

In this article, we summarized some experimental experience on this topic, mainly derived from studies in dogs, which leads us to the conclusion that the primary, direct effect of sympathetic coronary innervation is α-adrenergic coronary constriction, both in coronary resistance vessels and in the large, epicardial conductance arteries. In the resistance vessels, this neurogenic constriction is effectively counteracted by metabolic coronary dilation. In the large extramural conductance arteries, remote from myocardial cells and from their metabolic signals (e.g. adenosine), the neurogenic constriction is counteracted by an endothelium mediated, flow-dependent dilation [10, 11], which might be activated by changes in shear stress on the luminal surface of the endothelial cells.

Kupper, W. (ed.), Coronary tone in ischemic heart disease. ISBN 0-89838-646-2.
© *1984, Martinus Nijhoff Publishers, Boston/The Hague/Dordrecht/Lancaster. Printed in the Netherlands.*

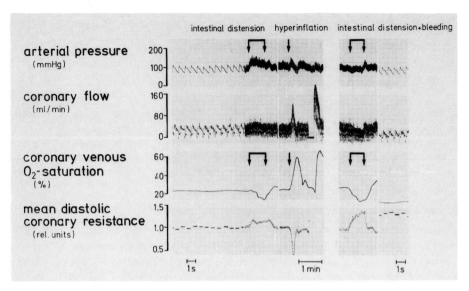

Figure 1. Modulation of coronary flow and of coronary venous oxygen extraction by reflexes in a conscious dog with experimental AV-block, no β-blockade was applied. Intestinal distension was induced by inflating a balloon chronically implanted in the small intestine. Hyperinflation of the lung by a deep inspiration was provoked by injecting 1.5 μg/kg nicotine into one carotid artery to stimulate the chemoreceptors. Following the decay of the hyperinflation induced coronary dilation, the coronary artery was occluded by an implanted cuff for zero flow control. When the increase in arterial pressure during intestinal distension was prevented by appropriate bleeding (right hand panel), a decline in coronary flow was observed (see high speed tracing). For calculation of mean diastolic coronary resistance, signals were replayed from magnetic tape at high speed for beat-to-beat calculation of the pressure–flow relation (from [38] by permission).

Reflexes directly modulating coronary flow

Experimental examples with direct sympathetic modulation of coronary flow and of coronary oxygen extraction in conscious dogs are shown in Figure 1. In these experiments, no β-blockade was applied; yet the heart rate was kept constant by ventricular pacing of the hearts, in which an AV-block has been produced previously by selective destruction of the bundle of His [12]. With this artificial constancy of heart rate, one major factor causing changes in myocardial metabolism and in extravascular coronary resistance during the activation of reflexes was eliminated. Thus, the analysis of direct nervous effects on the coronary vessels was simplified without affecting pharmacologically the possible interaction between coronary vascular β- and α-adrenoceptors.

In these conscious dogs, sympathetic activation by intestinal distension (inflation of a latex balloon chronically implanted in the small intestine) induced a relative coronary constriction and an increase in coronary oxygen extraction. This is indicated by the increase in mean diastolic coronary resistance and by the decrease in coronary venous oxygen saturation. The opposite reaction was elicited by the hyperinflation reflex (Figure 1). Certainly, intestinal distension does not result in a specific reflex reaction. This moderately irritating stimulus (inflation of the intestinal balloon) induced a nonspecific sympathetic activation, but was tolerated by the unrestrained, unsedated animals without any signs of discomfort and without any movements. The increase in arterial pressure observed during this sympathetic activation (Figure 1) was not the primary reason for the decline in coronary venous oxygen saturation: prevention of the increase in blood pressure by appropriate bleeding during intestinal distension unmasked the decline in coronary flow, while the decline in coronary venous oxygen saturation was even more pronounced (Figure 1).

The coronary dilation elicited by the pulmonary inflation reflex in dogs has been analyzed in detail by Vatner and McRitchie [13]. In conscious dogs, this coronary dilating reflex can be triggered by deep inspirations, which might occur spontaneously or can be induced by bolus injections of nicotine into one carotid artery [13]. In the dogs with constant heart rate, such a deep inspiration induces an increase in coronary flow, followed by a large increase in coronary venous oxygen saturation (Figure 1). This decline in coronary venous oxygen extraction demonstrates that the coronary dilation cannot result from increased myocardial metabolic demands, but is induced by direct actions of reflexes on the coronary vessels, independent of actions on myocardial metabolism. In Figure 2, this dilation is characterized pharmacologically. It is not modified by nonselective β-blockade or by muscarinic blockade, but is abolished by nonselective α-adrenergic blockade. Therefore, the dilation can be interpreted as a reflex withdrawal of sympathetic constriction. Similarly, nonselective α-blockade abolishes the coronary constriction induced by intestinal distension. Thus, in the conscious dog, the physiologic coupling between myocardial metabolism and coronary flow can be modulated substantially by increments or withdrawal of sympathetic α-adrenergic coronary control (Figure 3).

Pharmacologic α-blockade and sympathetic coronary constriction

The interpretation of coronary dilations being mediated by withdrawal of sympathetic constrictive control implies that a rather substantial α-adrenergic influence on the coronary resistance vessels exists in the conscious dog. However, nonselective α-blockade by phentolamine does not induce a coronary dilation with elevated coronary venous oxygen saturation (Figure 2). If the postulated constrictive coronary control existed, the pharmacologic removal of this control should result in a coronary dilation and in a decline in coronary oxygen extraction, but this cannot be observed. However, due to the complex central and peripheral effects of nonselective α-blockade in vivo, the existence of a con-

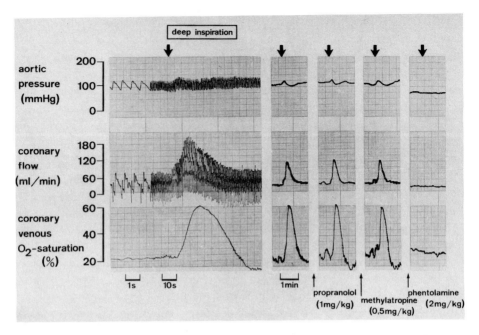

Figure 2. Pharmacologic characterization of the hyperinflation-induced coronary dilation in a conscious dog with AV-block. Arrows at the top of the record indicate a deep inspiration, provoked by injection of 1.5 μg/kg nicotine into a carotid artery. First panel: The deep inspiration causes a coronary dilation and a substantial increase in coronary venous oxygen saturation, indicating a hyperinfusion of the myocardium exceeding metabolic demands. Therefore, the dilation cannot be caused metabolically. Second panel: Same reaction as in the first panel, but coronary flow and arterial pressure are averaged electronically. Third and fourth panels: The dilation is not modified by β-adrenergic and by muscarinic blockade. Fifth panel: Alpha-adrenergic blockade by phentolamine abolishes the hyperinflation-induced coronary dilation (from [38] by permission).

strictive coronary control cannot be disproved by such an experiment.

Nonselective α-antagonists competitively block α_1- and α_2-adrenoceptors, the two constrictive subtypes which exist postsynaptically at vascular smooth muscle cells of many mammals including man [14–16]. Concomitantly, a strong sympathomimetic effect results from the α_2-component of nonselective α-blockade, by far exceeding the sympathetic activation due to reflexes. This effect is induced by central sympathoexcitation by α_2-blockade [17] and is amplified by the augmentation of action potential induced transmitter release from peripheral sympathetic nerve endings due to blockade of the presynaptic autoreceptors at these endings [18–20]. In the intact dog, this sympathoexcitation by nonselective α-blockade (at the dose applied in the experiments of Figure 2) results in a dramatic elevation of plasma catecholamines, strong activation of the renin-angiotensin system, increased total body oxygen consumption and β-adrenergic vasodilation [21, 22]. Comparison with selective α_2-blockade at equivalent dosage indicates that this strong signs of sympathoexcitation are not related to the induced changes in blood pressure [22]. When the metabolic and β-adrenergic vascular actions of this sympathoexcitation are suppressed by appropriate β-blockade, phentolamine does not lower the peripheral resistance in conscious dogs, though the vasoconstriction by exogenous norepinephrine is decreased 28-fold [21], and though peripheral resistance in these dogs is lowered substantially by selective $α_1$-blockade [21], which is devoid of sympathomimetic actions [23, 24], these studies demonstrate that the postsynaptic competitive vascular α-blockade in the intact organism might be almost compensated (or overcompensated, when selective $α_2$-blockade is applied, see [22] by the central and peripheral sympathoexcitation induced by this blockade. Therefore, unselective α-blockade cannot unmask the existence of an α-adrenergic constrictive control in a certain vascular bed of the intact organism.

Unfortunately, the same is true with selective $α_1$-blockade in vascular beds in which sympathetic constriction is mediated by activation of postsynaptic vascular $α_2$-adrenoceptors. With the identification of postsynaptic vascular $α_2$-adrenoceptors it was proposed that the vascular $α_1$-adrenoceptors are preferentially innervated, while the vascular $α_2$-adrenoceptors are extrasynaptically activated only by circulating catecholamines [25, 26]. However, this idea has been challenged recently by the demonstration of neurogenic, $α_2$-mediated vasoconstriction in several species [27–30]. In the canine coronary resistance vessels, both circulating [31] and neurogenic norepinephrine [32] appear to constrict the coronary bed mainly by activation of $α_2$-adrenoceptors. This explains why $α_1$-blockade in conscious dogs only transiently and variably dilates the coronary bed [33], but does not maintain a coronary dilation at a time, when full blockade of systemic $α_1$-adrenoceptor is demonstrable [33].

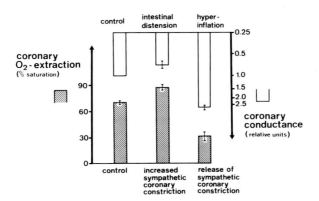

Figure 3. Modulation of the coupling between myocardial oxygen consumption and coronary flow by increased and decreased sympathetic coronary constriction in conscious dogs with constant heart rate (AV-block). Mean values ±SEM from ten experiments in five dogs. Intestinal distension and hyperinflation were induced as described in Figure 1.

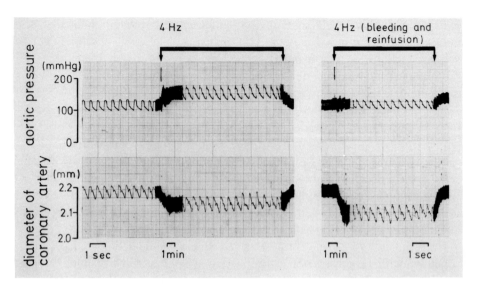

Figure 4. Constriction of coronary conductance artery in response to stimulation of the decentralized left stellate ganglion (arrows indicate duration of stimulation). Record from a dog in N_2O-pentobarbital anesthesia with constant heart rate (AV-block). The internal diameter of the circumflex branch of the left coronary artery is obtained by an induction angiometer. When the increase in arterial pressure during stimulation is minimized by appropriate bleeding, the decline in coronary artery diameter is more pronounced (from [38] by permission).

With nonselective or with α_2-selective blockade, the net effect between post-synaptic blockade and presynaptic and central augmentation of transmitter release should vary with the degree of sympathetic activity prior to the application of blockade. Actually coronary dilation with diminished coronary oxygen extraction can be induced by phentolamine in the exercising dog [34]. Probably, under this condition of high sympathetic activity, the transmitter release cannot be augmented much more, so that the postsynaptic blockade cannot be balanced completely. However, conclusions as to the degree of α-adrenergic constriction in an organ under physiologic conditions cannot be obtained from the application of α-adrenolytic drugs, when the constriction is mediated by activation of vascular α_2-adrenoceptors. (In experiments with anesthetized, spinalized animals with decentralized sympathetic ganglia, however, it is possible to suppress sympathetic vasoconstriction by α_2-blockade, since, under that condition, the strong central sympathoexcitation cannot play any role.)

In patients with frequent attacks of vasospastic angina pectoris, application of phentolamine (nonselective α-blocker) or prazosin (α_1-selective blocker) in controlled, double-blinded protocols did not attenuate the frequency or severity of attacks [35, 36]. The subtype of the human coronary vascular α-adrenoceptor is not identified, therefore, these studies cannot rule out completely the possibility of α-adrenergic constriction as the mechanism of coronary spasm in these patients (though other arguments militate against this possibility, see [8]).

Epicardial coronary conductance vessels and α-adrenergic constriction

The existence of functionally innervated α-adrenoceptors in epicardial coronary arteries has been documented by experiments under β-adrenergic blockade [37]. Under this condition, sympathetic nerve stimulation induces a moderate constriction of epicardial coronary arteries (Figure 4), but the degree of arterial narrowing is very small in the dogs with a healthy coronary system. Hemodynamically relevant coronary artery spasms cannot be elicited by sympathetic nerve stimulation.

In only one study was the effect of sympathetic stimulation on epicardial coronary arteries in situ analyzed without prior application of β-blockade [38]. In this study, the stimulation resulted in epicardial artery constriction, which was attenuated by phentolamine, thereby demonstrating that the primary effect of neurogenic norepinephrine on epicardial coronary arteries in situ is α-adrenergic constriction [38]. This is in contrast to an overwhelming number of studies in vitro, showing β-adrenergic coronary dilation as the primary effect of norepinephrine and of perivascular nerve stimulation (for review see [9]). It is not clear, what kind of preparative damage is responsible for this shift in the reactivity of isolated coronary smooth muscle in vitro away from the physiologic pattern of reaction in vivo.

The subtype of the postsynaptic vascular α-adrenoceptor on epicardial coronary arteries has not been identified exactly. Vatner et al. [39] observed a moderate epicardial artery constriction in conscious dogs induced by methoxamine, an α-adrenergic agonist with preferential action on α_1-adrenoceptors. Similarly, the coronary diameter at a defined arterial pressure was decreased slightly by methoxamine and increased by phentolamine in patients [40]. However, α_2-selective agonists were not applied for comparison in both studies. In isolated smooth muscle of canine epicardial coronary arteries in vitro, adrenergic constriction turned out to be mediated mainly by activation of α_1-adrenoceptors [41, 42]. It is a well-known experience that in studies on isolated vascular smooth muscle it is rather difficult to demonstrate α_2-mediated constrictions, which can be readily shown in in vivo studies. It is not clear whether this difference is the result of different localization of vascular α-adrenoceptors (α_1 predominating on the large arteries, which can be prepared for in vitro studies, while α_2-adrenoceptors are more frequent at the arterioles) or of changes in reactivity as a result of preparative damage. It was suggested recently that α_2-adrenoceptors exist additionally on endothelial cells [43]. The activation of these endothelial α_2-adrenoceptors triggers the release of an unidentified endothelial relaxing factor, thus counteracting the constriction resulting from activation of α_2-adrenoceptors on the smooth muscle cells [43]. It is possible that this mechanism contributes to the difficulties in demonstrating α_2-mediated constriction in arterial smooth muscle in vitro.

Endothelium mediated, flow-dependent dilation

In retrospect it is interesting to note that the sole study demonstrating sympathetic constriction of epicardial coronary arteries in situ without prior application of β-blockade was performed in a preparation, in which cornary flow did not increase during sympathetic nerve stimulation [38]. In this study, a blood perfused coronary artery at a non-working ventricle was analyzed, and the flow through this artery was constant. An increase in flow through an artery causes a dilation of this artery, as was shown for the first time 50 years ago by Schretzenmayer in the canine femoral artery [44]. At that time, a conduction of a dilatory signal from the arterioles to the arteries was proposed at the mechanism of this dilation, which was called 'ascending dilation.' Schretzenmayers observation was confirmed repeatedly, but later it was shown by a dissection experiment that ascending conduction could not be the mechanism of this dilation [45].

In isolated, perfused segments of canine coronary arteries with careful control of transmural pressure, it was shown recently that this flow-dependent dilation is abolished with removal or damage of the endothelium [10], while the response of these segments to directly acting constrictive or dilating stimuli was not modified. We propose that changes in flow through an artery cause changes in shear stress on the luminal surface of the endothelial cells, thus triggering the release of one or several endothelial factors causing dilation of the adjacent smooth muscle cells. This is a further example of endothelium-mediated dilation; similar dilations have been identified in the arterial response to acetylcholine by the pioneering studies of Furchgott's laboratory [46], and in the response to luminal hypoxia [47, 48] and to a number of drugs and hormones. In conscious dogs with chronic registration of epicardial artery diameter it could be demonstrated that there is a moment-to-moment regulation of epicardial coronary artery diameter by the flow rate through this endothelial mechanism [11]. This shear stress induced endothelial dilation is strong enough to convert the serotonin-induced constriction of epicardial coronary arteries in vivo into a dilation [49], when coronary flow is allowed to increase during serotonin application. Similarly, coronary flow increases substantially during stimulation of cardiac sympathetic innervation in experiments without β-adrenergic blockade. This metabolically induced increase in flow must have dilated the epicardial coronary arteries in previous studies by the endothelial mechanism, thereby preventing the α-adrenergic coronary constriction. This primary effect of the sympathetic coronary innervation could be observed only in Gerova's model of the non-working heart with constant flow [38]. It remains to be established whether this endothelium mediated, flow dependent dilation is operative in human vessels, too. It would be a protective mechanism against all kinds of constrictive stimuli acting on epicardial vessels. A loss of this protective mechanism by localized endothelial damage or a reduction of its influence during periods of low coronary flow at night might contribute to the localization of coronary spasms to circumscribed sites of the vessel and to their temporal predominance in the resting patient at night.

Conclusion

Functionally innervated α-adrenoceptors are documented both in large coronary conductance arteries and in coronary resistance vessels. The primary effect of sympathetic coronary innervation is α-adrenergic vasoconstriction in these two different vessel sections. In the coronary resistance vessels, metabolic dilation predominates, but the coupling between myocardial metabolism and coronary flow rate can be modulated by varying sympathetic coronary constriction. The amount of sympathetic constrictive coronary control cannot be evaluated by pharmacologic α-blockade due to its complex sympathomimetic actions. In the coronary conductance arteries, the α-adrenergic constriction is counteracted by factors such as a flow-dependent, endothelium-mediated dilation.

Acknowledgment

This research was supported by Dr-Karl-Wilder-Stiftung.

References

1. Kattus AA: Prinzmetal angina: Mechanisms, evaluation and management. Adv Heart Dis 1:245–251, 1977.
2. Maseri A: Pathogenetic mechanisms of angina pectoris: expanding views. Br Heart J 43:648–660, 1980.
3. Conti CR, Curry RC Jr: Coronary artery spasm and myocardial ischemia. Mod Conc Cardiovasc Dis 49:1–6, 1980.
4. Maseri A, Chierchia S: Coronary artery spasm: demonstration, definition, diagnosis, and consequences. Progr Cardiovasc Dis 25:169–192, 1982.
5. Rafflenbeul W, Lichtlen PR: Zum Knozept der 'dynamischen' Koronarstenose. Z Kardiol 71:439–444, 1982.
6. Bertrand ME, LaBlanche JM, Tilmant PY et al: Frequency of provoked coronary arterial spasm in 1089 consecutive patients undergoing coronary arteriography. Circulation 65:1299–1306, 1982.
7. Prinzmetal M, Kennamer R, Merliss R, Wada T, Bor N: Angina pectoris. 1: A variant form of angina pectoris. Am J Med 27:375–388, 1959.
8. Chierchia S: The role of alpha-adrenergic receptors in the pathogenesis of coronary spasm. Clin Cardiol 6:496–500, 1983.

52

9. Feigl EO: Coronary physiology. Physiol Rev 63:1–205, 1983.
10. Holtz J, Busse R, Giesler M: Flow-dependent dilation of canine epicardial coronary arteries in vivo and in vitro: Mediated by the endothelium. Naunyn-Schmiedebergs Arch Pharmacol 322:R44, 1983.
11. Holtz J, Giesler M, Bassenge E: Two dilatory mechanisms of antianginal drugs on epicardial coronary arteries in vivo: indirect, flow-dependent, endothelium-mediated dilation and direct smooth muscle relaxation. Z Kardiol (in press).
12. Von Restorff W, Bassenge E: Evaluation of a neurogenic rapid coronary dilation during an excitatory response in conscious dogs. Pflügers Arch 367:157–164, 1976.
13. Vatner SF, McRitchie RJ: Interaction of the chemoreflex and the pulmonary inflation reflex in the regulation of coronary circulation in conscious dogs. Circ Res 37:664–673, 1975.
14. Timmermans PBMWM, Van Zwieten PA: The postsynapic α_2-adrenoceptor. J Auton Pharmacol 1:171–183, 1981.
15. McGrath JC: Evidence for more than one type of post-junctional α-adrenoceptor. Biochem Pharmacol 31:467–484, 1982.
16. Elliot HL, Reid JL: Evidence for postjunctional vascular α_2-adrenoceptors in peripheral vascular regulation in man. Clin Sci 65:237–241, 1983.
17. McCall RB, Schuette MR, Humphrey SJ, Lahti RA, Barsuhn C: Evidence for a central sympathoexcitatory action of alpha-2 adrenergic antagonists. J Pharmacol Exp Ther 224:501–507, 1983.
18. Starke K: Regulation of noradrenaline release by presynaptic receptor systems. Rev Physiol Biochem Pharmacol 77:1–124, 1977.
19. Langer SZ: Presynaptic receptors and their role in the regulation of transmitter release. Br J Pharmacol 60:481–497, 1977.
20. Majewski H, Rump LC, Hedler L, Starke K: Effect of α_1- and α_2-adrenoceptor blocking drugs on noradrenaline release rate in anesthetized rabbits. J Cardiovasc Pharmacol 5:703–711, 1983.
21. Saeed M, Sommer O, Holtz J, Bassenge E: α-adrenoceptor blockade by phentolamine causes β-adrenergic vasodilation by increased catecholamine release due to presynaptic α-blockade. J Cardiovasc Pharmacol 4:44–52, 1982.
22. Saeed M, Holtz J, Sommer O, Kühne G, Bassenge E: β-adrenergic activation of the renin-angiotensin system following α_2-. α_1-, or nonselective α-blockade in conscious dogs: no relation to the changes in blood pressure. J Cardiovasc Pharmacol (submitted for publication).
23. Davey MJ: Relevant features of the pharmacology of prazosin. J Cardiovasc Pharmacol 2:287–301, 1980.
24. McCall RB, Humphrey SJ: Evidence for a central depressor action of postsynaptic α_1-adrenergic receptor antagonists. J Autonom Nerv Syst 3:9–23, 1981.
25. Langer SZ, Shepperson NB, Massingham R: Preferential noradrenergic innervation of alpha$_1$-adrenergic receptors in vascular smooth muscle. Hypertension 3:I-112–118, 1981.
26. Langer SZ, Shepperson NB: Recent developments in vascular smooth muscle pharmacology: the postsynaptic α_2-adrenoceptors. Trends Pharmacol Sci 3:440–444, 1982.
27. Gardiner JC, Peters CJ: Postsynaptic α_1- and α_2- adrenoceptor involvement in the vascular responses to neuronally released and exogenous noradrenaline in the hindlimb of the dog and cat. Eur J Pharmacol 84:189–198, 1982.
28. Wilffert B, Gouw MAM, De Jonge A, Timmermans PBMWM, Van Zwieten PA: Indications for vascular alpha- and beta-2 adrenoceptors in synapses of the muscarinic pathway in the pithed normotensive rat. J Pharmacol Exp Ther 223:219–223, 1982.
30. Elsner D, Saeed M, Sommer O, Holtz J, Bassenge E: Sympathetic vasoconstriction sensitive to α_2-adrenoceptor blockade: no evidence for preferential innervation of α_1-adrenoceptors in the canine femoral bed. Hypertension (submitted for publication).
31. Holtz J, Saeed M, Sommer O, Bassenge E: Norepinephrine constricts the canine coronary bed via postsynaptic α_2-adrenoceptors. Eur J Pharmacol 82:199–202, 1982.

32. Heusch G, Deussen A: The effects of cardiac sympathetic nerve stimulation on perfusion of stenotic coronary arteries in the dog. Circ Res 53:8–15, 1983.
33. Bassenge E, Holtz J: Sympathetic control of coronary circulation. In: Delius W, Gerlach E, Grobecker H, Kübler W (eds) Catecholamines and the Heart. Springer-Verlag, Berlin, 1981, pp 39–52.
34. Heyndrickx GR, Muylaert P, Pannier JL: α-adrenergic control of oxygen delivery to myocardium during exercise in conscious dogs. Am J Physiol 242:H805–809, 1982.
35. Chierchia S, Crea F, Davies G, Berkenboom G, Maseri A: Coronary spasm: any role for alpha-receptors? Circulation 66:II-47, 1982.
36. Winniford MD, Filipchuk N, Hillis LD: Alpha-adrenergic blockade for variant angina: a long-term, double-blind, randomized trial. Circulation 67:1185–1188, 1983.
37. Kelley KO, Feigl EO: Segmental alpha-receptor-mediated vasoconstriction in the canine coronary circulation. Circ Res 43:908–917, 1978.
38. Gerova M, Barta E, Gero J: Sympathetic control of major coronary artery diameter in the dog. Circ Res 44:459–467, 1979.
39. Vatner SF, Pagani M, Manders WT, Pasipoularides AD: Alpha adrenergic vasoconstriction and nitroglycerin vasodilation of large coronary arteries in the conscious dog. J Clin Invest 65:5–14, 1980.
40. Mishima M, Inoue M, Hori M, et al: The role of alpha-adrenergic activity in large and small coronary arteries in man. Circulation 66:II-153, 1982.
41. Cohen RA, Shepherd JT, Vanhoutte PM. Prejunctional and postjunctional actions of endogenous norepinephrine at the sympathetic neuroeffector junction in canine coronary arteries. Circ Res 52:16–25, 1983.
42. Rimele TJ, Rooke TW, Aarhus LL, Vanhoutte PM: Alpha-1 adrenoceptors and calcium in isolated canine coronary arteries. J Pharmacol Exp Ther 226:668–674, 1983.
43. Cocks TM, Angus JA: Endothelium-dependent relaxation of coronary arteries by noradrenaline and serotonin. Nature 305:627–630, 1983.
44. Schretzenmayer A: Über kreislaufregulatorische Vorgänge an den grossen Arterien bei der Muskelarbeit. Pflügers Arch Ges Physiol 232:743–748, 1933.
45. Lie M, Sejersted OM, Kiil F: Local regulation of vascular cross section during changes in femoral arterial blood flow in dogs. Circ Res 27:727–737, 1970.
46. Furchgott RF, Zawadzki JV: The obligatory role of endothelial cells in the relaxation of arterial smooth muscle by acetylcholine. Nature 288:373–376, 1980.
47. Busse R, Pohl U, Kellner C, Klemm U: Endothelial cells are involved in the vasodilatory response to hypoxia. Pflügers Arch Ges Physiol 397:78–80, 1983.
48. Busse R, Förstermann U, Matsuda H, Pohl U: The role of prostaglandins in the endothelium-mediated vasodilatory response to hypoxia Pflügers Arch Ges Physiol (in press).
49. Pohl U, Burger W, Holtz J, Bassenge E: Basis of ambivalent effects of serotonin and ergonovine on epicardial arteries in vivo. Circulation 68:II-32, 1983.

Discussion

Dr. Dickenson: I wonder if you have any information about the effect of indometacin or other similar drug on this reaction, because quite recently the group at Hammersmith Hospital reported enormous increases in circulating prostacycline during exercise, where flow is massively increased and one wonders whether such an effect could play any role in your experiments.

Dr. Bassenge: This was of course the first thing we were checking and the answer is: We do not see any changes of these reactions after indometacin.

Dr. McGregor: Surely you did not fail to see a vasodilatation.

Dr. Bassenge: No, after indometacin we observed the same changes in väsodilatation in this particular model.

Dr. McGregor: How did you administer it? Acutely?

Dr. Bassenge: Both. We administered it acutely, that means one hour before the experiments were started, and we administered it also about two hours before the dogs were sacrificed. You know that this is one-way-acetylation of the enzyme.

Dr. Vatner: Do you have any further thoughts on the seeming paradox between the large increases in coronary flow with respiration that are blocked by phentolamine and inability to demonstrate an increase in blood flow with either an alpha-blocker or with sympathectomy?

Dr. Bassenge: Well, I tried to point this out. I think it is impossible to demonstrate this by any pharmacological means, since both alpha-1 and alpha-2 receptors are present in the coronary bed. This means that you have to block both receptors. If one use an selective alpha-1 blocker, then the alpha-2 receptors remain sensitive in the preparation. If you administer phentolamine, which blocks both alpha-1 and alpha-2 receptors, then you block the autoinhibition of the transmitter release; hence you get an enormous increase in circulating norepinephrine due to the phentolamine administration, which causes an undefined competition between the blocking agent phentolamine and the excessively liberated norepinephrine on the vascular alpha receptors. That means, we get alpha-mediated changes in coronary resistance vessels, which we can not define accurately.

Dr. Vatner: But that does not explain, why with sympathectomy you don't see an increase in baseline flow, if the mechanism of this dilation is due to a release of alpha-tone.

Dr. Bassenge: This is true. We were able to show an increase in flow very quickly after chemical (6-Ohda) sympathectomy. The fast reduction with time of the excess flow after sympathectomy is probably due to some alteration in autoregulation after the sympathectomy. That means that other local control mechanisms take over, so that the sympathectomy is soon not effective anymore similar to the reaction observed in peripheral circulation: after sympathectomy you get a great increase in blood flow which disappears within one or two hours.

Dr. McGregor: The maneuver, which you call 'deep inspiration', is in anesthetized animals, isn't it? Is it forced inflation?

Dr. Bassenge: No, it can be elicited in unanesthetized animals. Dr. Vatner has described this in two papers. I think you can wait for a spontaneous deep breath of the animal, if the animal lies down and stretches. In addition you can experimentally induce this either by small amounts of nicotine injected into the area of the carotid bifurcation or by other means; you can also induce this by rapidly inflating the lungs in anesthetized preparations. But in a non-anesthetized preparation this reflex works much better and anesthesia is going to suppress this reflex almost completely, which has been shown by Dr. Vatner repeatedly.

Dr. McGregor: Most of the studies you talked about were in anesthetized dogs?

Dr. Bassenge: No, about 70% were done in conscious animals.

Dr. Dickenson: I was somewhat surprised that after intravenous adenosine administration you could not only demonstrate the well established increase in coronary artery flow but also in diameter. I always thought that adenosine dilates the peripheral resistance vessels rather than the conductance vessels. What is the explanation for this change in diameter?

Dr. Bassenge: Well, both is true. You can evoke a change in diameter of the epicardial coronary arteries by different drugs, for instance, administration of nitroglycerine dilates the coronary arteries without any increase in flow what so ever. This is one extreme on one side. Other drugs, like serotonine, cause arteriolar dilatation and cause an increase in blood flow and this increase in blood flow leads to a flow dependent increase in large vessel diameter. If you block this arteriolar dilatation, then serotonine becomes constrictive at the site of the large coronary arteries. So the flow-dependent dilatation is counteracted by the direct effect of serotonine on large coronary arteries resulting in a pronounced constriction of the large arteries. This is the other extreme. There are various drugs in between, like several calcium channel blockers, which have direct effects on the large coronary arteries in addition to the effects initiated by the flow dependent mechanism.

Dr. McGregor: This is a new thought to me, this flow-dependent increase in diameter. You have said: anything which increases the flow through a large vessel will by itself be a vasodilatator. You as well as Vatner have shown that postreactive hyperemia does dilate large coronary vessels and I think you gave me the reason, why we didn't find it: You have shown that it takes a long time to produce this flow dependent increase – your in vitro slides showed about a 8 min to get the peak effect. When we first studied this, we looked at large vessel resistance during reactive hyperemia and found no vasodilatation, but now I can see the reason why.

Dr. Vatner: We also showed that adenosine and dipyridamole dilate large coronary arteries. Several years ago we showed that a brief coronary occlusion resulted in a prolonged large coronary vasodilatation. We were able to block the response to a brief coronary occlusion completely by restriction of coronary flow, but we were unable to block completely the responses of large coronary arteries to acetylcholine or adenosine or to cardiac pacing. We were still able to demonstrate some vasodilation with these interventions even in the presence of constant coronary blood flow.

Dr. Bassenge: Well, I did not claim that this is the only mechanism for any sort of large epicardial vessel dilatation, but this is certainly one important mechanism. On top of that there might be metabolic mechanisms which you will probably discuss afterwards and which may be active via the pericardial fluid or something else. I do not know at present another mechanism for large coronary artery dilation.

Dr. Vatner: The other concern I have is that all the examples of flow related dilation of large arteries have almost always been demonstrated with very large increases in blood flow for example, five-fold increases in blood flow. Do you have any evidence that with very small increases or decreases of flow you can achieve similar results?

Dr. Bassenge: In our preparation in the conscious animal the increases were 2 to 4 times during post-occlusion hyperemia and were 2 to 3 times higher as basal flow in the experiments using adenosine,

Dr. Vatner: These are very large increases. Did you see anything, if blood flow changed less than 50%?

Dr. Bassenge: With small increases we cannot show the exact magnitude. We were glad that we were able to demonstrate this mechanism also with smaller flow increments ($\pm 20\%$); and we were able to show that the same happens in perfused segments of coronary arteries.

Dr. McGregor: Is this a new mechanism for second wind in anginal patients?

Dr. Bassenge: Yes, this is one hypothesis; it may be one explanation for the 'walk through angina' or also for various clinical observations like spasm occurring at 4 o'clock in the night, when flow, pressure, metabolism, etc. are very low. At such an occasion you would expect that the endothelial release of a dilating factor is minimal, and therefore, chances for an additional constriction of large epicardial coronary arteries is greatest. But I have to emphasize that these are only hypotheses, but they fit into the picture.

6. Regulation of large coronary arteries by beta adrenergic mechanisms in conscious dogs

STEPHEN F. VATNER & THOMAS H. HINTZE

Introduction

The goal of the present investigation was to test the hypothesis that large coronary arteries are regulated by beta $(\beta)_1$ adrenergic mechanisms and to determine by direct and continuous measurements, the extent to which activation of β_1 and β_2 adrenergic receptors elicited vasodilation of large and small coronary vessels in conscious dogs. This was accomplished by administering isoproterenol, an agent which contains β_1 and β_2 adrenergic properties, and pirbuterol, an agent which is thought to contain primarily β_2 adrenergic properties [25], in the presence and absence of selective β_1 adrenergic receptor blockade. Furthermore, selective β_1 adrenergic stimulation was accomplished with prenalterol, which does not possess β_2 stimulating properties [21]. The second goal of this investigation was to determine the mechanism of the constriction, which occurs after administering β_1 or α adrenergic receptor blockade. This involved determining whether the constriction was mediated by inhibition of β adrenergic tone and changes in myocardial metabolic demands or due to release of unopposed alpha (α) adrenergic tone. It was considered important to study this in conscious dogs, since anesthesia modifies autonomic control of the circulation [31], as well as vascular reactivity [2].

Methods

Mongrel dogs were anesthetized with pentobarbital Na, 30 mg/kg. Transducers were implanted through a thoracotomy in the 5th left intercostal space. Two miniature 7 MHz ultrasonic transducers (2×1 mm, 12 mg) were implanted on opposing surfaces of the left circumflex coronary artery, 3–6 cm from its origin. The ultrasonic transducers were covered with Insl-X (Insl-X Products Corp., Yonkers, NY) and attached to a Dacron (Dupont, de Nemours & Co., Inc., Wilmington, DE) backing. The Dacron was sutured to the outer adventitia of the coronary artery using Ethicon 6-0 suture (Ethicon, Inc., Somerville, NJ). An electromagnetic or Doppler flow transducer was implanted distally on the same

Kupper, W. (ed.), Coronary tone in ischemic heart disease. ISBN 0-89838-646-2.
© *1984, Martinus Nijhoff Publishers, Boston/The Hague/Dordrecht/Lancaster. Printed in the Netherlands.*

vessel. Pacing electrodes were implanted on the right atrium. Miniature pressure gauges (Konigsberg Instruments, Inc., Pasadena, CA) were implanted in the left ventricle and descending thoracic aorta and heparin-filled Tygon (Norton Co., Plastics and Synthetics Div., Tallmadge, OH) catheters were implanted in the left atrium and descending thoracic aorta. Coronary sinus catheters were implanted at a subsequent operation through a right thoracotomy approach after general anesthesia with pentobarbital Na, 25 mg/kg.

Left ventricular (LV) pressure was measured with the implanted miniature gauge, which was calibrated in vitro with a mercury manometer and cross calibrated in vivo with measurements of pressure from the aortic and left atrial catheters. Coronary blood flow was measured using a Benton square wave electromagnetic flowmeter (Benton Instruments, Cupertino, CA), or a Doppler ultrasonic flowmeter. Phasic coronary arterial diameter was measured instantaneously and continuously with an inproved ultrasonic dimension gauge [20, 26, 28, 32]. The frequency response of the dimension gauge is flat to 100 Hz. The drift of the instrument is minimal, i.e. less than 0.01 mm in 6 h. To further ensure data reliability, repeated calibration references were obtained regularly throughout the experiments, and the received ultrasonic signal was monitored continuously on an oscilloscope. Any major changes in alignment of the crystals was detected in the received signal and invalidated the experiment.

The experiments were conducted 1–3 weeks after operation in healthy conscious dogs lying quietly. Measurements of left circumflex coronary arterial diameter, aortic root pressure, LV pressure, LV dP/dt, LV diameter, left atrial pressure, left circumflex coronary blood flow, and heart rate were recorded continuously during control and interventions. The various interventions were carried out on different experimental days. Combined β_1 and β_2 adrenergic receptor stimulation was accomplished with i.v. bolus doses of isoproterenol, $0.1\,\mu g/kg$. Bolus doses of pirbuterol, $1.0\,\mu g/kg$, were also administered i.v. The $1.0\,\mu g/kg$ dose was selected to compare with the isoproterenol dose of $0.1\,\mu g/kg$, since pilot studies in which dose response curves were examined, demonstrated similar reductions in arterial pressure with these doses of the two drugs. After recovery from isoproterenol and pirbuterol, β_1 adrenergic receptor blockade was accomplished with i.v. atenolol (1.0 mg/kg), and isoproterenol ($0.1\,\mu g/kg$), and pirbuterol ($1.0\,\mu g/kg$) were administered again. The dose of atenolol was selected on the basis of its ability to block inotropic responses to isoproterenol without blocking peripheral vasodilator responses to isoproterenol. Atropine (0.1 mg/kg) was administered after β_1 adrenergic receptor blockade and isoproterenol ($0.1\,\mu g/$ kg), and pirbuterol ($1.0\,\mu g/kg$) were injected again. Then isoproterenol and pirbuterol were administered after combined β_1 and β_2 adrenergic receptor blockades with propranolol, 1 mg/kg. Selective β_1 adrenergic receptor stimulation was accomplished with prenalterol, $4,0\,\mu g/kg/min \times 5\,min$, for a total dose of $20\,\mu g/kg$, i.v. Due to the long half life of prenalterol [21], it was administered on separate days in the presence and absence of selective β_1 adrenergic receptor blockade. In the dogs with coronary sinus catheters experiments were conducted 1 week postoperatively, and samples of arterial and coronary sinus blood were drawn prior to and during peak responses to isoproterenol, pirbuterol, and prenalterol. Arterial and coronary sinus O_2 contents were measured using a LEX O_2 CON-K oximeter (Lexington Instruments, Lexington, MA). In the same dogs propranolol (0.5 mg/kg administered in two doses 5 min apart), which blocks β_1 and β_2 adrenergic receptors, and atenolol (0.5 mg/kg administered in 2 doses 5 minutes apart) which selectively blocks β_1 adrenergic receptors were administered on separate days. In other dogs blockade of α_1 and α_2 adrenergic receptors was achieved with phentolamine (2 mg/kg) followed by a continuous infusion (1 mg/min.). Then atenolol (1 mg/kg, or 0.5 mg/kg in two doses 5 min apart) was administered in the presence of phentolamine. The effects of 0.5 mg/kg of atenolol was indistinguishable from those of the 1.0 mg/kg dose. Prazosin was administered i.v., (1 mg/kg) to block α_1 adrenergic receptors, followed by atenolol, 1.0 mg/kg.

The data were recorded on a 14-channel tape recorder (Bell & Howell Co., Datatape Div., Pasadena, CA) and played back on two multichannel oscillographs (Gould-Brush, Cleveland, OH). Mean pressures and coronary diameters, and blood flows were assessed using RC filters with 2-s time constants. LV dP/dt was derived by differentiating the LV pressure signal using a Philbrick operational amplifier (Teledyne Philbrick, Dedham, MA), connected as a differentiator and having a frequency response of 700 Hz. A triangular wave signal with known slope (rate of change) was substituted for the pressure signal to calibrate the differentiator directly. Heart rate was measured continuously with a cardiotachometer triggered by the LV pressure pulse. While external coronary diameter was measured continuously, the internal radius was calculated by determining at autopsy the mass of a coronary artery with known length from the point at which the piezoelectric crystals were located. Thus, wall volume could be calculated as the quotient of mass and density (d = 1.06 g/cm³). After the wall volume, one wall thickeness value, and external diameter were known, the internal changing diameter was calculated.

Late diastolic coronary resistance, which reflects primarily small coronary vessel resistance was calculated as the quotient of late diastolic arterial pressure and late diastolic coronary blood flow. Mean and SEM were calculated for all variables. Data were analyzed before and after autonomic blockade using Student's t test for paired comparisons [3]. To adjust for the increased incidence of Type 1 errors consequent to double comparisons, the critical probability level was computed by the Bonferroni method [24], as the ratio of α/k, where α equals the error rate ($p<0.05$) and k equals the number of tests (n = 2). Thus, the critical possibility level of $p<0.025$ was utilized, when more than one comparison was examined.

Discussion

The effects of β adrenergic receptor stimulation have not been examined previously on direct and continuous measurements of large coronary arterial dimensions in the intact animal. The lack of information is due most likely to the absence of appropriate measuring techniques. Most prior studies have relied upon measurements of coronary blood flow and arterial pressure and calculations

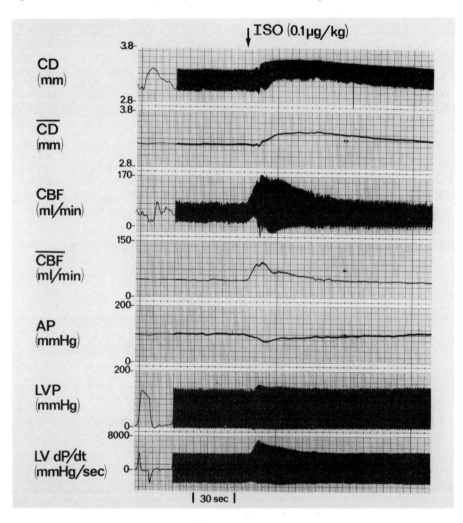

Figure 1. The effects in a conscious dog, of isoproterenol (ISO), 0.1 μg/kg, on measurements of phasic and mean left circumflex coronary diameter (CD), coronary blood flow (CBF), mean arterial pressure (AP), left ventricular pressure (LVP), and LV dP/dt. Shortly after isoproterenol was injected, peak effects were observed for arterial pressure, coronary blood flow, and LV dP/dt, while peak effects on coronary diameter occurred at a later point in time (reprinted with permission from Circulation Research).

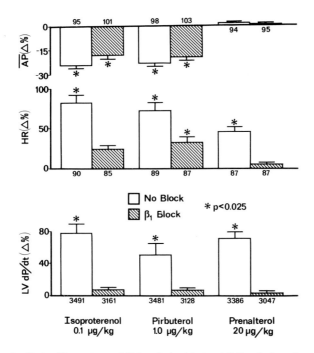

Figure 2. The peak effects of isoproterenol (0.1 μg/kg), pirbuterol (1.0 μg/kg), and prenalterol (20 μg/kg) are compared on percent changes in mean arterial pressure (AP), heart rate (HR), and LV dP/dt, before and after selective β₁-adrenergic receptor blockade with atenolol, 1.0 mg/kg. Baseline values are shown beneath the bars. Responses significantly different from control are noted by the symbols. Selective β₁-adrenergic receptor blockade did not alter responses of mean arterial pressure significantly, but attenuated responses of heart rate markedly and practically abolished inotropic responses (reprinted with permission from Circulation Research).

of coronary vascular resistance. These measurements assess primarily resistance coronary vascular responses. Recently we developed techniques to measure left circumflex coronary dimensions directly and continuously in conscious dogs [32]. The advantages and limitations in this methodology have been discussed in detail previously [20, 32]. Utilizing this methodology in the current investigation, we examined the extent to which large and small coronary arteries respond to β adrenergic receptor stimulation. Effects on small coronary vessels were assessed by calculations of late diastolic coronary vascular resistance, while effects on large coronary arteries were assessed by calculations of left circumflex coronary cross sectional area.

Isoproterenol increases myocardial O_2 consumption and consequently dilates resistance coronary vessels on a metabolic basis. In addition, isoproterenol also dilates coronary vessels by its action on vascular β adrenergic receptors [5, 17, 27, 35] independent of changes in myocardial metabolic demands. Most prior studies conducted in open-chest, anesthetized animals, indicate that isoproterenol stim-

62

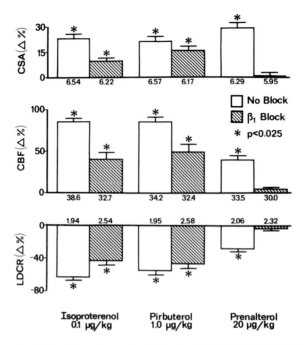

Figure 3. The peak effects of isoproterenol, pirbuterol, and prenalterol are compared on percent changes in coronary cross-sectional area (CSA), mean coronary blood flow (CBF), and late diastolic coronary vascular resistance (LDCR), before and after selective β_1-adrenergic receptor blockade with atenolol, 1.0 mg/kg. Baseline values are shown beneath the bars. Responses significantly different from control are noted by the symbols (reprinted with permission from Circulation Research).

ulation of vascular receptors in coronary resistance vessels is primarily β_2 mediated, since it still occurs after selective β_1 blockade [1, 13, 22, 23, 30]. An exception to this is the study by Lucchesi and Hodgeman [19], observing blunted coronary vascular as well as myocardial inotropic responses to β adrenergic receptor stimulation after selective β_1 adrenergic receptor blockade. It is also important to note the considerable evidence, which superficially appears contradictory, from studies in isolated coronary vessels, which would suggest that isoproterenol stimulates β_1 adrenergic vascular receptors [4, 7, 8, 16]. Since the latter studies examined primarily large coronary arteries, and whereas studies in open-chest anesthetized animals [1, 13, 22, 23, 30] assessed primarily effects on smaller, coronary resistance vessels, it is conceivable that both points of view are correct. One other point must be considered in understanding differences between experiments conducted in isolated vessels and more intact preparations. Until recently, it has generally been accepted that acetylcholine constricts isolated vessel preparations [9], but dilates coronary vessels *in vivo* [6, 18]. Recently Furchgott and Zawadzki [10] noted that these differences could be attributed to manipulation of the endothelium in isolated vessel preparations. It is also conceivable that β_2 adrenergic vascular receptors are located in the endothelial surface of large coronary arteries, and can only be demonstrated on isolated vessel preparations, if special care is taken not to disturb the endothelium.

As expected, in the present investigation, with β_1 and β_2 adrenergic receptors intact, isoproterenol induced a substantial reduction in calculated coronary vascular resistance. The drug also increased large coronary arterial cross-sectional area, which occurred at a later time than the peak increase in coronary blood flow, but still in the face of reduced arterial pressure (Figure 1). Since the decrease in pressure should have induced passive constriction of the large coro-

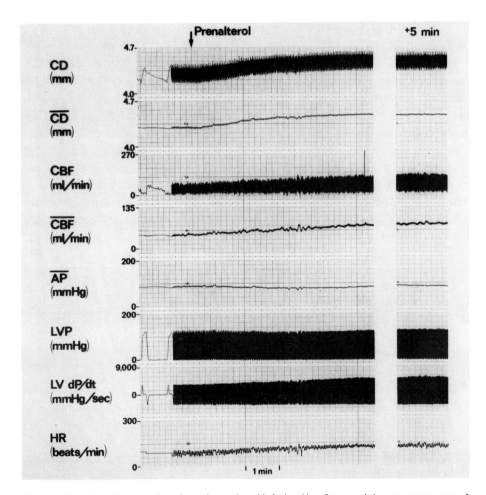

Figure 4. The effects in a conscious dog, of prenalterol infusion (4 μg/kg per min) on measurements of phastic and mean left circumflex coronary diameter (CD), coronary blood flow (CBF), mean arterial pressure (AP), LV pressure, LV dP/dt, and heart rate. The panel at right shows the peak effects 5 minutes after cessation of infusion. The increases in coronary diameter and blood flow occurred with prenalterol at similar points in time (reprinted with permission from Circulation Research).

nary vessels, the active dilation induced by isoproterenol was probably slightly underestimated.

If the isoproterenol induced vasodilation was simply due to β_2 adrenergic receptor stimulation, it should not have been affected by β_1 adrenergic receptor blockade. However, after selective β_1 adrenergic receptor blockade, iso-proterenol induced similar reductions in arterial pressure (indicating that pe-ripheral vascular β_2 adrenergic receptors were intact), but failed to increase LV dP/dt significantly (indicating that myocardial β_1 adrenergic receptors were essen-tially blocked) (Figure 2). Under these conditions, isoproterenol elicited signifi-cantly less dilation of both small and large coronary arteries (Figure 3). To eliminate the potential contribution of the tachycardia secondary to vagal with-drawal, experiments were repeated after combined β_1 adrenergic and cholinergic receptor blockades. Furthermore, with isoproterenol 0.1 μg/kg/min, heart rate was held constant after β_1 adrenergic receptor blockade. Under both these conditions isoproterenol failed to increase heart rate as well as LV dP/dt, but still reduced arterial pressure and dilated large coronary arteries. The effects on large coronary arteries, while significant, were markedly less than observed in dogs when heart rate rose.

The results of these experiments are compatible with the hypothesis that isoproterenol induces dilation of large coronary arteries not only by stimulation of vascular β_2 adrenergic receptors, but conceivably also by direct stimulation of vascular β_1 adrenergic receptors. The results are also consistent with the hypoth-esis that regulation of large as well as small coronary arteries occurs secondarily to changes in myocardial metabolism [20].

In order to stimulate β_2 adrenergic receptors primarily, we administered pir-buterol [25]. Dose response curves indicated that a 1.0 μg/kg dose of pirbuterol elicited an equivalent reduction in arterial pressure to a 0.1 μg/kg dose of iso-proterenol. We were surprised to find that the responses to pirbuterol and isoproterenol were so similar in terms of effect not only on the coronary circula-tion, but also on LV dP/dt and heart rate (Figures 2 and 3). In part the similarity between the two agents can be ascribed to secondary reflex effects on heart rate and myocardial contractility.

In order to selectively stimulate β_1 adrenergic receptors, prenalterol was ad-ministered (Figure 4). The selectivity of this agent in terms of stimulating β_1 adrenergic receptors in the conscious dog has been noted previously in our laboratory [21]. While it has been reported that prenalterol may exert other actions, e.g., β_2 adrenergic blocking effects under some experimental conditions [14, 33], it is important to note that we observed no effect of the drug after selective β_1 adrenergic blockade. Thus, any action of prenalterol, other than of β_1 adrenergic receptor stimulation is not of great importance under the conditions of the present experiments. In these experiments, prenalterol, by stimulating β_1 adrenergic receptors, increased heart rate and LV dP/dt. These changes occurred over a similar time course with the decreases in calculated late diastolic coronary

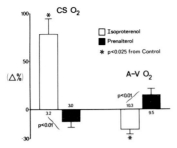

Figure 5. The effects of isoproterenol (open bars), pirbuterol (shaded bars), and prenalterol (solid bars) are compared on measurements of coronary sinus O_2 content (CSO$_2$) and A-V O_2 difference. Baseline values are shown beneath the bars. Isoproterenol and pirbuterol increased CS O_2 content and decreased A-V O_2 content difference. Prenalterol had the opposite effect.

vascular resistance and increases in large coronary arterial cross-sectional area (Figure 4). These experiments lend further support of the conclusion that the large coronary vessels dilate not only in response to β_2 adrenergic receptor stimulation, but also in response to either increases in myocardial metabolic demands [20], or to direct stimulation of β_1 adrenergic vascular receptors [4, 7, 8, 16].

To discern between primary vascular effects secondary to changes in myocardial metabolism, coronary sinus O_2 content and A-V O_2 content difference were measured (Figure 5). As was observed previously by Klocke et al. [17] in the current experiments isoproterenol either in the presence or absence of selective β_1 adrenergic receptor blockade induced excess coronary blood flow, increases in coronary sinus O_2 content, and reductions in A-V O_2 difference. We observed similar responses with pirbuterol. In contrast, prenalterol increased A-V O_2 difference slightly. Thus, it is likely that the additional β_2 adrenergic receptor stimulation induced by isoproterenol or pirbuterol activated β_2 vascular receptors and caused dilation of small and large coronary vessels independent of changes in myocardial O_2 demand. In contrast, the component of large vessel coronary dilation due to direct β_1 adrenergic receptor stimulation or secondary to β_1 adrenergic receptor stimulation of myocardial resistance vessels, was not of sufficient magnitude to elicit excess coronary blood flow, an increase in coronary sinus O_2 content and narrowing of A-V O_2 difference.

In view of the potential role of β adrenergic mechanisms in mediating vasospasm of large coronary arteries and the recent reports suggesting that vasospastic angina is exacerbated by propranolol [29] it was considered important to determine the effects of β adrenergic receptor blockade on large coronary arteries. The results of the present investigation indicate that propranolol, which blocks β_1 and β_2 adrenergic receptors, induces modest constriction of large coronary arteries in the conscious dog. Several possible mechanisms for the propranolol induced constriction of the large coronary arteries were considered:

(1) blockade of β_2 vasodilator tone, (2) a direct effect of propranolol on the coronary arteries, (3) predominance of unopposed α adrenergic tone, (4) blockade of β_1 effects and concomitant reduction in myocardial metabolic demands.

If the mechanism involved blockade of β_2 adrenergic receptor vasodilator tone, then atenolol, which selectively blocks β_1 adrenergic receptors, should not evoke the constriction. In fact, the results of this study, demonstrating constriction with atenolol suggest that the major mechanism of the coronary vasoconstriction involves blockade of β_1 adrenergic tone. It is important to note that the dose of atenolol used, 0.5–1.0 mg/kg, is sufficient to block β_1 adrenergic receptors, but does not block the depressor and vasodilator effects of isoproterenol.

One prevalent theory explaining the constriction of coronary arteries following

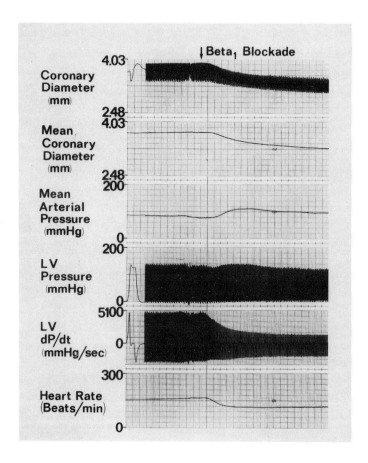

Figure 6. The effects of β_1-adrenergic blockade (atenolol) in the presence of α-adrenergic blockade (phentolamine) are shown in a conscious dog on measurements of phasic and mean left circumflex coroary arterial diameter (CD), arterial pressure (AP), left ventricular pressure (LVP), LV dP/dt, and heart rate. Administration of the β-adrenergic receptor blocker produced significant left circumflex coronary arterial constriction (reprinted wth permission from Circulation Research).

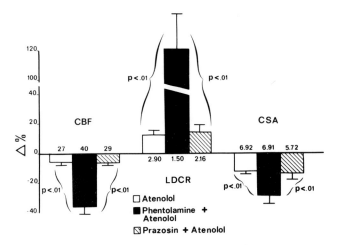

Figure 7. Effects of atenolol alone (open bars), atenolol in the presence of phentolamine (solid bars), and atenolol in the presence of prazosin (shaded bars), are compared as percent change from baseline for coronary blood flow (CBF), late diastolic coronary resistance (LDCR), and left circumflex coronary cross-sectional area (CSA). In the presence of phentolamine, atenolol produced greater constriction of resistance as well as large coronary arteries, compared with the similar effects observed in the absence of α-adrenergic receptor blockade and in the presence of selective α_1-adrenergic receptor blockade with prazosin (reprinted with permission from Circulation Research).

administration of β adrenergic receptor blockers is that α adrenergic tone becomes unopposed and consequently α vasoconstriction predominates [27]. To test this hypothesis, the β adrenergic receptor blockers were administered after blockade of α adrenergic receptors. Under these conditions if release of unopposed α adrenergic tone was important, then the vasoconstrictor effects of the β adrenergic receptor blocking agents would be eliminated, or at least diminished. This was not observed. In fact, the constriction of resistance coronary arteries as reflected by measurements of LDCR, as well as the constriction of large coronary arteries as reflected by reductions in CSA, was augmented significantly. The enhanced constriction was most likely due to the markedly elevated levels of norepinephrine and epinephrine observed after phentolamine. It is well recognized, and found in the study as well, that phentolamine blocks α_2 in addition to α_1 adrenergic receptors thereby causing enhanced levels of circulating catecholamines [12].

Recently, we noted that large coronary arteries are responsive to changes in myocardial metabolic demands, i.e. either increases in heart rate or ventricular wall tension induces dilation of large coronary arteries [20]. The results of the current investigation are compatible with these concepts. In the intact, resting conscious dog, β adrenergic receptor blockade induced only modest depression of heart rate and myocardial contractility, and concomitantly elicited only modest constriction of large coronary arteries. In the presence of phentolamine, β

68

adrenergic blockade elicited striking reductions in heart rate and myocardial contractility and consequently elicited more intense constriction of large coronary arteries as well as coronary resistance vessels (Figures 6 and 7). Under these conditions, when heart rate was held constant, and only myocardial contractility fell with the β adrenergic receptor blocking agent, the constrictor effects on the resistance and large coronary arteries were less marked. These observations are consistent with the concept that large coronary arteries are responsive to changes in myocardial metabolic demands. The mechanism by which a change in myocardial metabolic demand might influence large coronary arterial dimensions is not known. While it is known that adenosine concentration in the pericardial fluid varies with metabolic activity in the heart, this method of transmission of a metabolic message is unlikely, since the pericardium was incised widely at operation and not repaired. Another consideration is that the large coronary arteries are regulated by changes in coronary blood flow, as has been proposed by Gerova et al. [11]. We have recently observed that the reactive dilation of large coronary arteries secondary to brief periods of coronary occlusion and myocardial ischemia can be totally prevented by preventing the reactive hyperemia upon release of the coronary occlusion, whereas the increase in large coronary arterial dimensions secondary to increasing heart rate or adenosine administration are only partially attenuated [15].

In summary, the results of the present investigation indicate an important role for regulation of large coronary arteries by β adrenergic mechanisms. While in the normal heart the contribution of large coronary arteries to total coronary vascular resistance is small, about 5% [34], its role in the presence of myocardial ischemia, particularly due to partial occlusion of a large coronary artery, assumes greater significance where changes in large vessel calibre may be crucial in regulation of the flow to the ischemic area. β_1, as compared with β_2, adrenergic receptor stimulation appeared to exert more important effects on large coronary arteries. However, a role for β_2 adrenergic receptor stimulation was also demonstrated. It is conceivable that the β_1 adrenergic effects were secondary to changes in myocardial metabolism and not due to direct activation of specific β_1 vascular receptors. These conclusions must be tempered by the fact that these experiments were carried out with pharmacologic activation of β adrenergic receptors. Thus, the role of β adrenergic receptor regulation of large coronary arteries by neural activation remains to be demonstrated.

Summary

The effects of β adrenergic stimulation were examined in conscious dogs on measurements of left circumflex coronary arterial diameter and blood flow and on calculations of late diastolic coronary resistance (LDCR) and left circumflex coronary internal cross sectional area (CSA). Isoproterenol (0.1 μg/kg) initially decreased mean arterial pressure by $25 \pm 2\%$ (Mean $\pm$ SEM), and LDCR by $62 \pm 4\%$, and increased heart rate by $82 \pm 10\%$, left ventricular (LV) dP/dt by $79 \pm 12\%$, and mean coronary blood flow by $85 \pm 5\%$, while CSA rose slightly. The peak effects on CSA ($24 \pm 2\%$) occurred later, along with decreases in mean arterial pressure ($7.4 \pm 1.0\%$) and LDCR ($25 \pm 5.3\%$) and increases in coronary blood flow ($14 \pm 2\%$), LV dP/dt ($12 \pm 3\%$), and heart rate ($24 \pm 4\%$). Pirbuterol ($1.0\,\mu g/kg$) induced qualitatively similar changes to those of isoproterenol. Prenalterol ($20\,\mu g/kg$), a cardio-selective β_1 adrenergic receptor agonist, did not affect mean arterial pressure, but increased heart rate by $40 \pm 5\%$, LV dP/dt by $72 \pm 10\%$, mean coronary blood flow by $34 \pm 11\%$, CSA by $26 \pm 3\%$, and decreased LDCR by $29 \pm 5\%$. Isoproterenol and pirbuterol, but not prenalterol, increased coronary sinus O_2 content and decreased A-V O_2 difference. After β_1 adrenergic receptor blockade with atenolol ($1\,mg/kg$), prenalterol no longer induced significant effects, while isoproterenol and pirbuterol decreased mean arterial pressure similarly to what was observed prior to blockade, but did not increase LV dP/dt, and induced attenuated increases in mean coronary blood flow, CSA, and decreases in LDCR. Thus, in the intact, conscious animal large coronary arteries are regulated by β adrenergic mechanisms. Surprisingly, a major fraction of large coronary arterial dilation appeared to be either directly or indirectly due to β_1 adrenergic receptor mechanisms, although β_2 adrenergic effects were also significant. To determine the role of β adrenergic mechanisms in the constriction which results from administration of β_1 adrenergic blockade, the β_1 adrenergic blocker atenolol was administered after α adrenergic blockade with phentolamine. In the presence of alpha blockade, β_1 adrenergic receptor blockade induced even greater constriction of large coronary arteries. Thus, the dilation of large and small coronary arteries appears either directly or indirectly dependent upon β_1 adrenergic mechanisms.

Acknowledgment

This research was supported by USPHS Grants HL15416 and HL17459.

References

1. Adam KR, Boyles S, Scholfield PC: Cardio-selective β adrenoceptor blockade and the coronary circulation. Br J Pharmacol 40:534–536, 1970.
2. Altura BT, Altura BM: Pentobarbital and contraction of vascular smooth muscle. Am J Physiol 229:1635–1640, 1975.
3. Armitage P: Statistical Methods in Medical Research. Blackwell Scientific Publications, New York, 1973, pp 116–126.
4. Baron GD, Speden RN, Bohr DF: Beta-adrenergic receptors in coronary and skeletal muscle arteries. Am J Physiol 223:878–881, 1972.

70

5. Berne RM, Rubio R: Coronary circulation. In: Geiger SR (ed) Handbook of Physiology, sec 2. The Cardiovascular System, vol 1. American Physiological Society, Bethesda, Md, 1979, pp 873–952.

6. Blesa MI, Ross G: Cholinergic mechanisms on the heart and coronary circulation. Br J Pharmacol 38:93–105, 1970.

7. De La Lande IS, Harvey JA, Holt S: Response of the rabbit coronary arteries to autonomic agents. Blood Vessels 11:319–337, 1974.

8. Drew GM, Levy GP: Characterization of the coronary vascular β-adrenoceptor in the pig. Br J Pharmacol 46:348–350, 1972.

9. Furchgott RF: The pharmacology of vascular smooth muscle. Pharmacol Rev 7:183–265, 1955.

10. Furchgott RF, Zawadzki JV: The obligatory role of endothelial cells in the relaxation of arterial smooth muscle by acetylcholine. Nature 288:373–376, 1980.

11. Gerova M, Gero J, Barta E, Dolezel S, Smiesko V, Levicky V: Neurogenic and myogenic control of conduit coronary artery: a possible interference. Basic Res Cardiol 76:503–507, 1980.

12. Graham RM, Stephenson WH, Pettinger WA: Pharmacological evidence for a functional role of the prejunctional alpha-adrenoreceptor in noradrenergic neurotransmission in the conscious rat. Naunyn-Schmiedebergs Arch Pharmacol 311:129–138, 1980.

13. Gross GJ, Feigl EO: Analysis of coronary vascular beta receptors in situ. Am J Physiol 228:1909–1913, 1975.

14. Hedberg A, Mattson H, Carlsson E: Prenalterol, a non-selective β-adrenoceptor ligand with absolute β_1-selective agonist activity. J Pharm Pharmacol 32:660–661, 1980.

15. Hintze TH, Vatner SF: Reactive dilation of large coronary arteries in conscious dogs. Circ Res (in press).

16. Johannson B: The β-adrenoceptors in the smooth muscle of pig coronary arteries. Eur J Pharmacol 24:218–224, 1973.

17. Klocke FJ, Kaiser GA, Ross J Jr, Braunwald E: An intrinsic adrenergic vasodilator mechanism in the coronary vascular bed of the dog. Circ Res 16:376–382, 1965.

18. Levy MN, Zieske H: Comparison of the cardiac effects of vagus nerve stimulation and of acetylcholine infusions. Am J Physiol 216:890–897, 1969.

19. Lucchesi BR, Hodgeman RJ: Effect of 4-(2-hydroxy-3-isopropylaminopropoxy) acetanilide (AY 21,011) on the myocardial and coronary vascular response to adrenergic stimulation. J Pharmacol Exp Ther 176:200–211, 1971.

20. Macho P, Hintze TH, Vatner SF: Regulation of large coronary arteries by increases in myocardial metabolic demands in conscious dogs. Circ Res 49:594–599, 1981.

21. Manders WT, Vatner SF, Braunwald E: Cardio-selective beta-adrenergic stimulation with prenalterol in the conscious dog. J Pharmacol Exp Ther 215:266–270, 1980.

22. Mark AL, Abboud FM, Schmid PG, Heistad DD, Mayer HE: Differences in direct effects of adrenergic stimuli on coronary, cutaneous, and muscular vessels. J Clin Invest 51:279–287, 1972.

23. McRaven DR, Mark AL, Abboud FM, Mayer HE: Responses of coronary vessels to adrenergic stimuli. J Clin Invest 50:773–778, 1971.

24. Miller RG: Simultaneous Statistical Inference. New York, McGraw-Hill, 1966, pp 67–70.

25. Moore PF, Constantine JW, Barth WE: Pirbuterol, a selective β_2 adrenergic bronchodilator. J Pharmacol Exp Therap 207:410–418, 1978.

26. Pagani M, Vatner SF, Baig H, Franklin DL, Patrick T, Manders WT, Quinn P, Sherman A: Measurement of multiple simultaneous small dimensions and study of arterial pressure dimension relations in conscious animals. Am J Physiol 235:H610–H617, 1978.

27. Parratt JR: Effects of adrenergic activators and inhibitors on the coronary circulation. In: Szekeres (ed) Handbook of Experimental Pharmacology, vol. 54/I. Springer-Verlag, Berlin-Heidelberg, 1980, pp 735–822.

28. Patrick TA, Vatner SF, Kemper WS, Franklin D: Telemetry of left ventricular diameter and pressure measurements from unrestrained animals. J Appl Physiol 37:276–281, 1974.

29. Robertson RM, Wood AJJ, Vaughn WK, Robertson D: Exacerbation of vasotonic angina pectoris by propranolol. Circulation 65:281–285, 1982.

30. Ross G, Jorgensen CR: Effects of cardio-selective beta adrenergic blocking agent on the heart and coronary circulation. Cardiovasc Res 4:148–153, 1970.

31. Vatner SF, Braunwald E: Cardiovascular control mechanisms in the conscious state. N Engl J Med 293:970–976, 1975.

32. Vatner SF, Pagani M, Manders WT, Pasipoularides AD: Alpha adrenergic vasoconstriction and nitroglycerin vasodilation of large coronary arteries in the conscious dog. J Clin Invest 65:5–14, 1980.

33. Wagner RJ, Schumann HJ: The lack of a pronounced preference of prenalterol for the beta-1-adrenoceptor subtype. Naunyn-Schmiedebergs Arch Pharmacol 315:85–88, 1980.

34. Winbury MM, Howe BB, Hefner MA: Effect of nitrates and other coronary dilators on large and small coronary vessels: an hypothesis for the mechanism of action of nitrates. J Pharmacol Exp Ther 168:70–95, 1960.

35. Zuberbuhler RC, Bohr DF: Responses of coronary smooth muscle to catecholamines. Circ Res 16:431–440, 1965.

Discussion

Dr. Bassenge: How do the large epicardial coronary arteries know what is going on in the myocardium far behind in terms of metabolism? There must be something which connects both over a wide diffusion gap.

Dr. McGregor: Do you have any thoughts on how the metabolic demand status of the myocardium could influence the conductive vessels?

Dr. Vatner: One explanation might be that there is a liberation of adenosine into the pericardial fluid which might influence the large epicardial conductive vessels. Furthermore, part of the mechanism may be related to the flow phenomenon Dr. Bassenge presented. But we still observe some large coronary arterial vasodilation with pacing when blood flow is held constant.

Dr. Bassenge: Your pericardial hypothesis could be easily checked by removing the pericardium, so that there would be no possibility for a vasodilating substance to act via the pericardial fluid!

Furthermore, an additional question: was there any increase in flow, which was not paralleled by an increased metabolism in your experiments?

Dr. Vatner: I believe that some of the increases in coronary flow occurred above and beyond the increases in metabolism induced by isoproterenol and pirbuterol, since there was an excess of coronary sinus oxygen concentration. This was also observed with other vasodilators, for example nitroglycerine, acetylcholine, dipyridamole and adenosine.

Dr. Bassenge: So it remains to be clarified, how much is metabolically induced and how much is flow dependent.

Dr. Vatner: Yes. That is why I asked you before, whether you have investigated situations with very small changes in coronary flow. The flow dependent phe-

72

nomenon can be demonstrated with reactive dilation when 3–4-fold increases in coronary blood flow occur.

Dr. McGregor: Is there no evidence that adenosine acts on large vessels in a situation where flow and pressure are not varied, for instance in the isolated large vessel?

Dr. Vatner: Yes, there is some evidence that isolated large vessels do dilate in response to dipyridamole.

Dr. Bassenge: Using strips one can show a great variety of reactions. With strips one can specify pharmacological reactions, but their vasomotion is different from in vivo conditions.

Dr. Vatner: What we did, is to give a bolus of adenosine before and after holding flow constant. We were able to demonstrate about 1/3 of the large coronary vasodilator response remained intact.

Dr. McGregor: Inspite of the fall in coronary perfusion pressure!

Dr. Chierchia: You said that the response in diameter after reactive hyperemia is delayed and lasts for longer. Have you tried to correlate these changes with the changes in contractility usually happening after reactive hyperemia or a short period of occlusion?

Dr. Vatner: In our experiments during coronary occlusions of 10 to 30 seconds the only hemodynamic changes observed are very slight decreases in LV dp/dt. We do not see changes in arterial pressure and heart rate. In the experiments with constant coronary blood flow there are no hemodynamic changes and no reactive hyperemia during the recovery period. The effects on coronary blood flow generally occur very early.

We studied the effect of coronary occlusion with the occluder either proximal or distal to the crystals, which measured the dimension. If the occluder was proximal to the crystals a decrease in coronary dimensions occurred during occlusion. If the occluder was distal a slight rise occurred during occlusion. The peak effects occurred about 60 seconds after release and it required several minutes to recover. But at the peak time, after 60 seconds, there was no effect on the small resistance vessels and on hemodynamics.

Dr. Chierchia: What happened to the coronary artery diameter after beta-blockade during pacing?

Dr. Vatner: We see increases in coronary diameter when heart rate increases in the presence or absence of beta-blockade.

Dr. Chierchia: When you give beta-blockers, the diameter goes down quite dramatically, doesn't it?

Dr. Vatner: In our normal conscious dogs coronary diameter goes down very slightly, because these dogs don't have very much resting sympathetic tone. A beta-blocker administered to a normal dog decreases heart rate, approximately 5 to 7 beats per minute and decreases LV dp/dt on the order of 10%. Thus we observe only a small fall in coronary diameter with no change or a slight increase in arterial distending pressure of about 3 mmHg.

Dr. Mishima: What do you think about the beta-2-regulation of the epicardial coronary arteries?

Dr. Vatner: We think that there is beta 2-control of the large coronary arteries as well as the resistance vessels. We think that it is not regulated by neural mechanisms, but that these receptors can be activated by circulating catecholamines or by the administration of isoproterenol or pirbuterol. Our most surprising finding was that a significant fraction appears to be related to beta-mechanisms. Right now we are going one step further, looking at receptors in large coronary arteries using ligand binding techniques.

Dr. Dickenson: You have shown one slide where it was apparently that coronary artery diameter is not completely passively related to distending pressure. In particular, it seemed to be related to atrial contraction, wasn't it?

It is reminiscent of these funny little atrial waves, which have been reported over many years in peripheral arteries. Using this as a genuine effect, if so, might it be locally regulated, perhaps by atrial receptors or is it just some movement artefact? Were you able to rule that out? It is a phenomenon, which seems to depend on having an animal in a good condition, preferably not anesthetized. I have never quite understood whether this phenomenon is an artefact or a genuine tip of an ice-berg.

Dr. Vatner: We don't see this in peripheral arteries.

Dr. Dickenson: But it has been seen from others.

Dr. McGregor: There is something quite similar in man, an atrial kick in the peripheral arterial wave. Is it an artefact or have you any explanation?

Dr. Vatner: We don't. We don't know, whether it's due to motion of the heart. The timing of its appearance is co-incident with atrial systole.However, we were unable to rule out whether it was due to a change in cardiac motion or to an actual effect on coronary diameter.

Dr. Bassenge: We were able to demonstrate that already small decreases in flow ($\pm 20\%$) cause a decrease in liberation of this dilating factor. It is quite impressive that a brief occlusion by a cuff of only 3 to 5 seconds already tends to decline the large coronary arterial diameter proximal to the cuff.

7. The role of alpha-adrenergic activity in large and small coronary arteries in man

MASAYOSHI MISHIMA, MICHITOSHI INOUE, MASATSUGU HORI, TAKASHI SHIMAZU, HIROSHI ABE, KAZUHISA KODAMA & SHINSUKE NANTO

Introduction

Experimental studies [1–3] have shown that coronary artery vasoconstriction and increase in coronary vascular resistance can be elicted by sympathetic stimulation. Some clinical reports [4–7] have strongly suggested that in patients with variant angina alpha-adrenergic stimulation could induce clinical episodes of coronary spasm, whereas alpha-adrenergic blockade could be effective in alleviating these episodes. Thus, the alpha-adrenergic nervous system is regarded as one of several possible mechanisms that cause abnormal augmentation of coronary vasomotor reactivity. However, the physiological significance of alpha-adrenergic activity in regulation of coronary vascular tone is not well understood. In this study, we examined to what extent alpha-adrenergic stimulation with methoxamine and alpha-adrenergic blockade with phentolamine altered the coronary vascular tone, mainly the vascular tone of epicardial large coronary arteries.

Method

Patients (Table 1)

The study was performed on 17 patients undergoing cardiac catheterization because of a known or suspected coronary artery disease. These patients were divided into three groups. Five patients with chest pain syndrome and two patients with inferior myocardial infarction were subjected to the study for methoxamine (group 1, 7 men). Five patients with chest pain syndrome and one patient with inferior myocardial infarction (group 2, 5 men and 1 woman) were subjected to the study for phentolamine. Another four patients (group 3, 4 men) were administered ergonovine maleate in order to compare the effects of ergonovine maleate with those of the changes in alpha-adregenic activities on coronary vascular tone. None of the patients had significant coronary lesion, more than 50% in left coronary arteries.

Kupper, W. (ed.), Coronary tone in ischemic heart disease. ISBN 0-89838-646-2.
© 1984, Martinus Nijhoff Publishers, Boston/The Hague/Dordrecht/Lancaster. Printed in the Netherlands.

Table 1. Subjects in this study undergoing cardiac catheterization because of a known or suspected coronary artery disease

	No. of patients	M:F	Age
Methoxamine study			
chest pain syndrome	5	7:0	52 ± 6
inferior MI	2		
Phentolamine study			
chest pain syndrome	5	5:1	51 ± 5
inferior MI	1		
Ergonovine study			
chest pain syndrome	4	4:0	48 ± 5

Procedures

After routine right and left heart pressure measurements by femoral approach, a triple thermister thermodilution pacing catheter (Wilton Webster Laboratories, Altadena, CA) was inserted into coronary sinus with the distal thermister advanced to the great cardiac vein. Each patient was paced 15–20% above the basal sinus rhythm by arterial pacing throughout the study. Great cardiac venous flow (continuous thermodilution method) and cardiac output (thermodilution) were determined with aortic pressure measurement. Total peripheral resistance (TPR) as an index for systemic vascular tone was also obtained as follows:

$$\text{TPR (resistance unit)} = \text{mAP (mmHg)}/\text{CO (l/min)} \times 1/60,$$

where mAP and CO represent mean aortic pressure and cardiac output respectively. Then, magnified left coronary arteriogram (see below) by femoral ap-

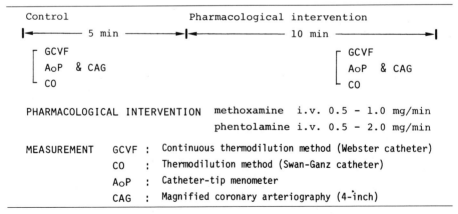

Figure 1. Protocol of this study: GCVF = great cardiac venous flow; CO = cardiac output; AoP = aortic pressure; CAG = coronary arteriography.

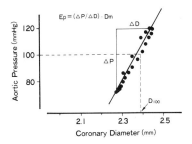

Figure 2. Representative pressure–diamter relationships of the left anterior descending coronary artery. The pressure–diameter relationships during a cardiac cycle showed a narrow clockwise loop. In the present study we determined the inclination of the loop and the diameter at 100 mmHg of aortic pressure in the descending limb to assess the vascular tone. Abbreviations: EP = dynamic incremental elastic modulus ($10^6 \cdot N \cdot m^{-2}$); D100 = coronary diameter at 100 mmHg of aortic pressure (mm); ΔP & Δ = difference of aortic pressure and coronary diameter between peak systole and end-diastole; Dm = mean coronary diameter.

proach was obtained in right anterior oblique position with simultaneous pressure measurement in sinus of Valsalva, using a catheter-tip manometer (Millar PC-481). At least 10 min after these control measurements, methoxamine (0.5–1.0 mg/min) or phentolamine (0.5–2.0 mg/min) was infused at a constant rate and maintained; aortic pressure increased (by methoxamine) or decreased (by phentolamine) by about 20 mmHg for about 10 min. Thereafter, the same measurements as the control were repeated to assess the effects of the alpha-adrenergic interventions (Figure 1).

In patients of group 3, at least 10 min after the control measurements, ergonovine maleate (0.1 mg i. v. at 3 min/intervals upto 0.4 mg) was administered, and same the measurements were performed as on groups 1 and 2.

In the present study, Ca^{2+}-antagonists, long acting nitrates and β-blockers, which could modify the coronary vascular tone, were not administered for at least 3 days before catheterization.

Pressure–diameter relationship of the large coronary arteries

Magnified coronary arteriography, using a 4-in. image intensifier, was performed with special care to keep the same projection angle and table-to-image intensifier distance. The measurements of the coronary arterial caliber from magnified coronary arteriograms were performed by the computerized image processing system, which has already been developed [8–10]. This system enabled us to obtain the pressure–diameter relationship of the large coronary arteries in vivo (Figure 2). The sampling site for caliber measurement was in the proximal left anterior descending coronary artery (LAD) 5–10 mm distal from the bifurcation.

78

Indices for evaluating coronary vascular tone

For the assessment of large coronary vascular tone, we obtained two indices of vascular wall distensibility. One is a dynamic incremantal elastic modulus, Ep(dyn), defined as follows [10, 11]:

$$Ep(dyn) = (\Delta P/\Delta D) \cdot Dm \ (10^{-6} \cdot N \cdot m^{-2}),$$

where ΔP and ΔD represent the pulse pressure and corresponding pulse diameter, respectively, and Dm is a mean diameter during a cardiac cycle (Figure 2). Another index is the absolute caliber at 100 mmHg of aortic pressure, D100 (Figure 2). Here, augmented vascular tone results in an increase in Ep(dyn) and in contrast a decrease in D100.

On the other hand, for the assessment of the vascular tone of small coronary arteries, resistance vessels, the regional coronary vascular resistance (RCVR)

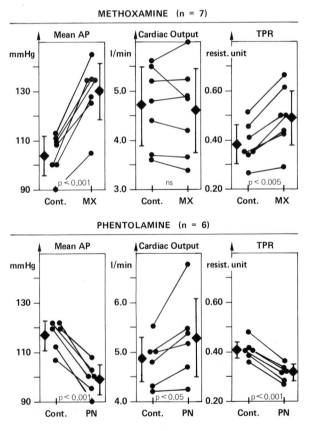

Figure 3. Effects of methoxamine i.v. and phentolamine i.v. on systemic hemodynamics. Abbreviations: AoP = aortic pressure; TPR = total peripheral resistance; Cont. = Control; MX and PN = methoxamine and phentolamine, respectively.

was determined from mean aortic pressure (mAP) and great cardiac venous flow (GCVF)

$$RCVR = mAP/GCVF \quad (mmHg/ml \cdot m^{-1})$$

Thus, the coronary vascular tone was assessed in large and small coronary arteries in LAD territory.

Statistical analysis

The statistical significance of the differences was determined using appropriate t-tests. When multiple group comparisons were made, a one way analysis of variance was performed. A p value of 0.05 or less was considered significant. All results in this study are expressed as mean ± standard devation.

Results

Effects of alpha-adrenergic interventions on systemic hemodynamics (Figure 3)

By infusion of methoxamine (0.5–1.0 mg/min; total 4–11 mg, in average 6.1 ± 2.3 mg) mean aortic pressure (104 ± 7.5 → 130 ± 11.6 mmHg) increased significantly by 24 ± 6.2% (p<0.001), but cardiac output (4.68 ± 0.78 → 4.60 ± 0.85 l/min) did not change (ns) and, thus, total peripheral resistance (0.384 ± 0.026 → 0.491 ± 0.115 resistance unit) increased significantly by 27% (p<0.001). In contrast, phentolamine (0.5–2.0 mg/min; total 5–18 mg, in average 11 ± 4 mg) decreased mean aortic pressure (117 ± 5.9 → 99 ± 5.7 mmHg) significantly by 15.2% (p<0.001) and cardiac output increased (4.83 ± 0.45 → 5.30 ± 0.80 l/min, p<0.005). Thereby the total peripheral resistance (0.407 ± 0.033 → 0.313 ± 0.034 resistance unit) decreased significantly (by 22.0%, p<0.01) similar to that of methoxamine.

   Thus we could change the systemic vascular tone, defined as total peripheral resistance, in the opposite direction to the same extent by methoxamine and phentholamine.

Effects of alpha-adrenergic interventions and ergonovine maleate on the large coronary arteries (Figure 4, Table 2)

By methoxamine, mean coronary diameter, Dm, did not change (3.34 ± 0.61 → 3.31 ± 0.59 mm, ns) despite a significant increase in aortic pressure, resulting in a significant decrease in coronary diameter at 100 mmHg of aortic pressure, D 100, (3.33 ± 0.61 → 3.23 ± 0.60 mm, p<0.05) and in significant increase in dynamic

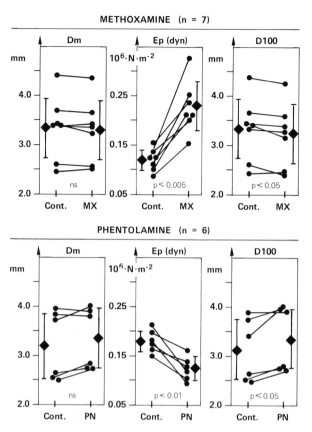

Figure 4. Effects of methoxamine i.v. and petholamine i.v. on large coronary artery. Abbreviations are the same as in Figures 2 and 3.

incremental elastic modulus, Ep (dyn), $(0.12 \pm 0.02 \rightarrow 0.23 \pm 0.05 \ 10^6 \cdot N \cdot m^{-2}$, p<0.01). These results indicated that the vascular tone in the large coronary arteries could be significantly increased by alpha-adrenergic stimulation. In contrast, by phentolamine, D100 increased significantly $(3.12 \pm 0.60 \rightarrow 3.35 \pm 0.60$, p<0.01) and Ep decreased $(0.18 \pm 0.02 \rightarrow 0.12 \pm 0.02$, p<0.01). Then it was also demonstrated that the vascular tone in the large coronary arteries could reduced by alpha-adrenergic blockade with phentolamine.

Ergonovine maleate raised aortic pressure significantly but caused minimal change in coronary diameter as well as methoxamine (Table 2). No localized vasospasm was observed. But D100 reduced significantly in all cases, demonstrating the augmentation of coronary vascular tone (p<0.01). The extent of these vasoconstrictive effects was much greater than that of methoxamine in spite of smaller vasoconstrictive effects on systemic arteries.

Effects of alpha-adrenergic intervention on the small coronary arteries (Figure 5)

During methoxamine infusion, great cardiac venous flow decreased in one patient but increased slightly the other six patients, resulting in a slight but insignificant increase in coronary vascular resistance ($2.12 \pm 0.63 \rightarrow 2.36 \pm 0.68$ mmHg/ml $\cdot$ min^{-1}).

Phentolamine caused no significant decrease in great cardiac venous flow in spite of a significant decrease in aortic pressure, resulting in significant decrease in coronary vascular resistance ($2.41 \pm 0.48 \rightarrow 2.16 \pm 0.49$ mmHg/ml $\cdot$ min^{-1}).

These results suggest that alpha-adrenergic tone could also modulate the vascular tone of small coronary arteries even under the autoregulation.

Discussion

The present clinical study demonstrated the significant effects of alpha-adrenergic interventions on coronary vascular tone, especially large coronary arterial tone, in man. Although the extent of those effects was less than those on the systemic resistance arteries and, in addition, those of ergonvine maleate on the large coronary arterial tone, this regulatory mechanism could be related to the pathophysiological mechanism of coronary spasm (Figure 6).

Previously the physiologic or pathophysiologic role of alpha-adrenergic ac-

*Table 2.*Changes in coronary diameters and dynamic incremental elastic moduli after administration of ergonovine maleate

Patient number	Age/sex	Aortic pressure				LAD			
		Cont		EM		Cont		EM	
		syst (mmHg)	diast (mmHg)	syst (mmHg)	diast (mmHg)	Ep(dyn) $10^6 \cdot$ N $\cdot$ m^{-2}	D100 (mm)	%ΔEp (%)	%ΔD100 (%)
1	43M	135	103	155	106	0.13	3.13	$-$ 8.3	$-$ 8.3
2	44M	130	85	143	86	0.17	3.35	20.2	$-$ 13.5
3	49M	115	75	145	83	0.23	2.37	$-$ 5.4	$-$ 13.8
4	56M	120	76	146	82	0.08	1.86	44.0	$-$ 32.8
mean	48	126	85	147	89	0.15	2.68	12.6	$-$ 17.3
SD	5	9	11	5	10	0.06	0.60	21.2	9.3

Abbreviations: LAD = left anterior descending coronary artery; Cont = Control; EM = ergonovine maleate; syst and diast = systole and diastole, respectively; Ep(dyn) = dynamic incremental elastic modulus; D100 = coronary diameter at 100 mmHg aortic pressure.

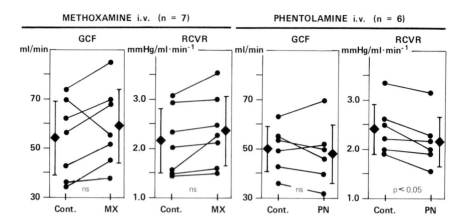

Figure 5. Effects of methoxamine i.v. and phentolamine i.v. on small coronary artery. Abbreviations: GCV flow = great cardiac venous flow; RCVR = regional coronary vascular resistance; other abbreviations are found in Figure 3.

tivities has been studied clinically on the basis of coronary caliber measurements, but the concomitant changes in aortic pressure were left out of consideration. The findings presented in this paper are unique in that the effects of vasoactive drugs on large coronary arteries were examined from the view point of the pressure–diameter relationship to avoid the influence of the changes in aortic pressure, i.e. coronary distending pressure (Figure 7). We used a computerized image processing system, which we had recently developed, to measure the coronary caliber from a magnified coronary arteriogram [8–10]. The changes in vascular tone in large coronary arteries were assessed by calculations of D100 and Ep(dyn),

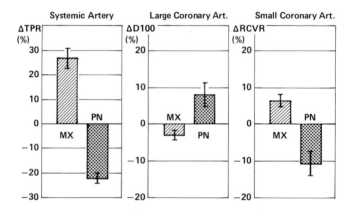

Figure 6. Effects of methoxamine i.v. and phentolamine i.v. on systemic and coronary arteries. Abbreviations are the same as in Figures 2 and 3.

whereas those in small coronary arteries were assessed by calculations of regional coronary vascular resistance. Thus, we could evaluate quantitatively the extent to which large and small coronary arteries respond.

For alpha-stimulation methoxamine was used, and phentolamine was used for alpha-blockade. Responses to ergonovine maleate were also investigated for comparison. It was considered that effects of either alpha-stimulation or alpha-blockade were incomplete. Vatner et al. [3] reported in their experimental study that methoxamine (50 μg/kg/min) raised mean aortic pressure by 65% and in-duced reductions in coronary diameter (by 9%). In our study less dosis of methoxamine (total 6.1 ± 2.3 mg) was infused slowly for more than 10 min. Although the increases in mean aortic pressure in our study (21%) were much less than that in their study, a significant increase in total peripheral resistance was observed in all patients, indicating the achievement of substantial alpha-stimula-tion. For alpha-blockade Macho et al. [12] administered in their experimental study a bolus dose of 2 mg/kg phentolamine followed by an infusion 0.1 mg/kg/min, inducing decreases in mean aortic pressure of approximately 20%. In our study less dosis of phentolamine (11.6 ± 5.4 mg) was administered, achieving substantially similar decreases (15.2%) in mean aortic pressure. Moreover, pre-vious clinical studies indicated that alpha-blockade can be achieved by 5–10 mg of phentolamine and could lead a relief of coronary spasm [4–7].

Another limitation is probable beta-adrenergic stimulation due to phentol-

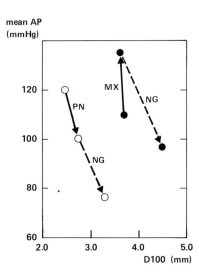

Figure 7. Effects of vasoactive drugs on large coronary arteries. Phentolamine and nitroglycerin caused coronary vasodilation in spite of the reduction in mean aortic pressure, as coronary distending pressure. In contrast to phentolamine and nitroglycerin, methoxamine induced coronary vasocon-striction against the elevation of mean aortic pressure. Abbreviations: PN, MX & NG = phen-tolamine, methoxamine & nitroglycerin, respectively.

*Table 3.*Changes in systemic and coronary hemodynamics, coronary diameters, and dynamic incremental elastic moduli during administration of phentolamine with β-blockade (propranolol)

	Control						PN with β-blockade			
	HR	mAP	TPR	RCVR	D100	Ep (dyn)	%Δ TPR	%Δ RCVR	%Δ D100	%Δ Ep
KM	70	98	0.327	1.63	2.74	0.22	−17.8	−22.7	+3.6	−16.1
ST	80	138	0.849	2.23	3.53	0.48	−29.4	−14.4	+4.8	−26.3

Abbreviations: HR = heart rate; mAP = mean aortic pressure; other abbreviations the same as in Table 2 and Figure 3.

amine-induced release of norepinephrine, which may cause concomitant of coronary vascular tone [3, 13, 14]. To evaluate to what extent such beta-stimulation contributes to the alteration of coronary vascular tone, the effects of phentolamine were further examined in two patients after beta-blockade (Table 3). In these two patients 5 mg of propanolol was administered intravenously 10 min before the control measurements, and the same measurements as group 2 were performed. In these patients, the reduction in total peripheral resistance (11.8% and 29.4%) was similar to that in group 2. Under such a condition, the effects of phentolamine on D100 (+3.6% and +4.8%) and on regional coronary vascular resistance (−22.7% and −14.4%) were found to be comparable to those of phentolamine without beta-blockade. These results indicated that the beta-stimulation due to phentolamine-induced release of norepinephrine contributes minimally to the alteration of coronary vascular tone.

In this study, alpha-adrenergic interventions are suggested to affect also the autoregulatory mechanism of small coronary arteries. However, considerable measurements may be derived from the concomitant changes in extravascular factors that affect the calculated regional coronary vascular resistance (RCVR). We evaluated the changes in vascular tone of small coronary arteries totally during a cardiac cycle, utilizing RCVR as an index, which was calculated as follows:

$$RCVR = mAP/GCVF.$$

Thus defined, RCVR could not reflect the sensitive changes in vascular tone of small coronary arteries. The genuine effects of alpha-adrenergic interventions on human small coronary arteries remain to be elucidated.

References

1. Schwartz PJ, Stone HL: Tonic influence of the sympathetic nervous system on myocardial reactive hyperemia and coronary blood flow distribution in dogs. Circ Res 41:51–58, 1977.

2. Mohrmann DE, Feigl EO: Competition between sympathetic vasoconstriction and metabolic vasodilation in the canine coronary circulation. Circ Res 42:79–86, 1978.
3. Vatner SF, Pagani M, Manders WT, Pasipoularides AD: Alpha-adrenergic vasoconstriction and nitroglycerin vasodilation of large coronary arteries in the conscious dog. J Clin Invest 65:5–14, 1980.
4. Yasue H, Touyama M, Shimamoto M, Kato H, Tanaka S, Akiyama F: Role of autonomic nervous system in the pathogenesis of Prinzmetal's variant form of angina. Circulation 50:534–539, 1974.
5. Yasue H, Touyama M, Kato H, Tanaka S, Akiyama F: Prinzmetal's variant form of angina as a manifestation of alpha-adrenergic receptor-mediated coronary artery spasm: documentation by coronary arteriography. Am Heart J 91:148–155, 1976.
6. Levene DL, Freeman MR: Alpha-adrenoceptor-mediated coronary artery spasm. JAMA 236:1018–1022, 1976.
7. Ricci DR, Orlick AE, Cipriano PR, Guthaner DF, Harrison DC: Altered adrenergic activity in coronary artery spasm: insight into mechanism based on study of coronary hemodynamics and the electrocardiogram Am J Cardiol 43:1073–1079, 1979.
8. Yachida M, Ikeda M, Tsuji S, Inoue M, Hori M, Shimazu T: Computer analysis of cine angiograms. Automedica 3:121–129, 1980.
9. Inoue M. Hori M, Inada H, Kitabatake A, Takeda H, Mishima M, Shimazu T, Kosuoka H, Abe H, Kodama K, Nanto S, Koretsune Y: Computerized assessment of coronary arterial pressure–diameter relationship in man. Effects of nitroglycerin and ergonovine maleate. Proceedings of World Congress on Medical Physics and Biomedical Engineering, 1982, 2.08, 1982.
10. Hori M, Inoue M, Shimazu T, Mishima M, Kusuoka H, Abe H, Kodama K, Nanto S: Clinical assessment of coronary arterial elastic properties by the image processing of coronary arteriograms. IEEE (in press).
11. Gow BS, Hadfield GD: The elasticity of canine and human coronary arteries with reference to postmortem changes. Circ Res 45:588–594, 1979.
12. Macho P. Hintze TH, Vatner SF: Effects of alpha-adrenergic receptor blockade n coronary circulation in consious dogs. Am J Physiol 243:H94–H98, 1982.
13. Doxey JC, Smith CFC, Walker JM: Selectivity of blocking agents for pre-and postsynaptic alpha-adrenoceptors. Brit J Pharmacol 60: 91–100, 1977.
14. Holz J. Saeed M. Sommer O, Bassenge E: Norepinephrine constricts the canine coronary bed via postsynaptic alpha 2-adrenoceptors. Eur J Pharmacol 82:199–202, 1982.

Discussion

Dr. Vatner: What happened to the heart rate or contractility with the phentolamine administration?

Dr. Mishima: (1) Heart rate was fixed by arterial pacing throughout the study. Every patient was paced 10–20% above the baseline sinus rhythm. (2) About contractility we cannot say anything. Phentolamine increased cardiac output, but this effect was probably influenced by the reduction in afterload.

Dr. Bassenge: How much did pressure fall after phentolamine administration and β-blockade?

Dr. Mishima: It was about 20 mmHg.

Dr. Bassenge: Did you perform any oxygen saturation measurements at the time the catheters in great cardiac vein and in the aorta were in place? What did you see after administration of methoxamine or phentolamine?

Dr. Mishima: Yes, we did. After methoxamine coronary A-VO$_2$ difference had a tendency to increase, but not significantly. Whereas after phentolamine we found a small but significant decrease in coronary A-VO$_2$, difference.

Dr. Mac Alpin: I had not previously been aware of anybody being able to demonstrate arteriographically pulsatile diameter changes in the human coronary arteries. I'm not surprised that they are there. Did your technique use a magnified angiogram with an automatic edge detection system? What orders of magnitude of pulsatile diameter changes did you see, what was the range?

Dr. Mishima: Yes, we had an magnified angiogram with computerized image processing system. The change in the caliber of left anterior descending coronary arteries during a cardiac cycle was $4.5 \pm 1.2\%$, up to 8%.

Dr. Mac Alpin: I have noticed that you did not see any of the presystolic changes that were seen in the animal models using ultrasound crystals.

Dr. Mishima: We could not detect it with our system.

Dr. Vatner: I think that there is a difference in frequency response of the two systems.

Dr. Mac Alpin: Considerable, I'm sure. But also the aberration was quite huge too.

Dr. Bassenge: An 8% pulsatile diameter change of the coronary arteries seems rather high, we see changes in the order of 1%.

Dr.Serruys: (1) We have tried to do the same things and we even tried it in patients during balloon-pumping. In these patients with or without balloon-pumping there was sometimes a difference in perfusion pressure throughout diastole of 30, even 45 mmHg. Even in these extreme situations we were unable to demonstrate a significant change in diameter greater than 0.2 mm which is quite close to the resolution of all available techniques. (2) Another point is, if you want to do frame-by-frame analysis of diameter of the coronary system there are two problems. There is always some kind of rotation of the coronary artery during the systole and diastole and this is one of the major problems especially if there is a coronary lesion. (3) With beginning of the ejection you have a fast motion of the coronary system and that is likely to induce some blurring effect.

Dr. Mishima: (1) With the magnified coronary arteriogram we could detect such changes in the magnitude above mentioned. (2) We hypothesized that the normal human epicardial coronary artery is round. Therefore, the tortion movement does not influence our measurements theoretically. (3) The coronary artery images were recorded on 35-mm cine films at a rate of 60 frames per second, and inner diameters of coronary arteries were obtained every two frames of coronary arteriogram. As you pointed, during arterial contraction we also found a fast motion, that may cause blurring effect. It is of very short duration and, just before the ejection, coronary arterial motion is not so fast. Therefore, we found no difficulties to obtain pressure-diameter loops in our patients.

Dr. McGregor: We should avoid equating large and small vessels with those vessels that are conductive and those that are metabolically autoregulated. I say that for the following reason. If you introduce vasoactive materials by injecting them with xenon in saline straight into the muscle, all materials I have ever tested except methoxamine produced the expected effect. Vasoconstrictors reduced the washout of xenon and vasodilators did the opposite. That is to say drugs were introduced to the microvasculature while bypassing the conductive vessels. Methoxamine introduced in that way, however, did not have any effect by contrast with its potent effect when it passes through the length of the coronary arteries. This makes me think you are showing us the effect of changes of tone of large vessels and possibly quite small conductive vessels, which have an effect on resistance. But these are not necessarily the same vessels that are metabolically autoregulated.

Dr. Mishima: As I defined in my paper, we evaluated the changes in coronary vascular tone using pressure–diameter relationship for large epicardial coronary artery, proximal LAD, and regional coronary vascular resistance for small coronary arteries. From the pressure–diameter relationship we can estimate the effects of interventions on the proximal LAD as a representative of large vessels. On the other hand, by coronary vascular resistance, the changes in tone of resistance vessels are totally evaluated. There may be conductive small vessels and also other small vessels autoregulated metabolically, as you said. In my paper, we did not differentiate those.

8. Adrenergic control of human coronary circulation

G.H. MUDGE, JR. & PETER GANZ

There is mounting clinical evidence to suggest that coronary artery vasoconstriction may be important in provoking intermittent myocardial ischemia in patients with coronary artery disease. The alpha-adrenergic nervous system may be potential physiologic mediator of such inappropriate coronary artery vasoconstriction. Animal studies have documented that tonic alpha-adrenergic mediated vasoconstriction tone exists both at rest and with exercise [1–3]. Carotid sinus nerve stimulation or the administration of phentolomine, an alpha-adrenergic blocking agent, reduces this tonic coronary artery vasoconstrictor activity. Resting alpha-adrenergic vasoconstrictor tone has also been demonstrated in the human coronary circulation [4]. Orlick and co-workers compared the resting coronary hemodynamics in patients with normally innervated hearts to those with denervated hearts following cardiac transplantation. With similar myocardial metabolic demands, those patients with denervated hearts had a higher coronary blood flow and lower coronary vascular resistance at rest when compared to a normal population. When phentolomine was administered intravenously, those patients with denervated hearts had a fall in coronary blood flow that paralleled a fall in coronary perfusion pressure, in contradistinction to the normal innervated population in which a fall coronary perfusion pressure was associated with an increase in coronary blood flow. This indicates that basal alpha-adrenergic coronary vasoconstrictor tone is a determinant of resting coronary artery blood flow.

Inappropriate coronary artery vasoconstriction has been observed in patients with coronary artery disease during the alpha-adrenergic stimulation of cold exposure. This observation has been documented by measuring coronary blood flow with both the coronary sinus thermodilution technique and Xenon 133 images [5, 6]. Such alpha-adrenergic stimulus has not been documented to cause significant change in the diameter of the epicardial coronary arteries, although some observes have used this stimulation to provoke coronary artery spasm [7]. It has been postulated that the coronary artery vasoconstrictor effect occurs at the level of the small resistance vessels; patients with significant coronary artery disease may have maximal or near-maximal vasodilation at the arteriolar level, and hence, a superimposed vasoconstrictor stimulus is associated with a fall in coronary artery blood flow [5]

Kupper, W. (ed.), Coronary tone in ischemic heart disease. ISBN 0-89838-646-2.
© *1984, Martinus Nijhoff Publishers, Boston/The Hague/Dordrecht/Lancaster. Printed in the Netherlands.*

Beta-adrenergic blockade with propranolol has been reported to intensify both the duration and degree of myocardial ischemia in patients with coronary artery spasm [8]. Recent investigations have documented that acute intravenous beta-adrenergic blockade can increase the adrenergically mediated vasoconstrictor response to the cold pressor test [9]. It is postulated that beta-adrenergic blockade inhibits bate-2 mediated vasodilatory mechanisms, hence leaving alpha-adrenergically mediated vasoconstriction unopposed. Such inappropriate vasoconstriction can be abolished by the administration of phentolomine, a pre- and post-synaptic (alpha-2 and alpha-1, respectively) alpha-adrenergic blocking agent. Such general alpha-adrenergic blockade might result in enhanced circulating norepinephrine levels due to blockade of the presynaptic alpha-2 receptor (receptors which inhibit the release of norepinephrine). It was speculated that selective post-synaptic alpha-1 blockade might inhibit coronary artery vasoconstriction due to cold exposure, without inducing potentially deleterious effects of nonselective alpha-adrenergic blockade. Accordingly, the purpose of a recently completed investigation by Kern et al. [10] at the Brigham and Women's Hospital was to test the hypothesis that selective alpha-1 adrenergic blockade might attenuate the inappropriate reflex increase in coronary vascular resistance due to alpha-adrenergic stimulus without increasing the circulating levels of norepinephrine.

Eleven patients undergoing diagnostic catheterization with classic anginal discomfort were initially evaluated. Patients were excluded who had left main coronary artery disease, severe left ventricular dysfunction. unstable angina, or coexistant valvular heart disease. Patients were also excluded who were on nonsteroidal antiinflammatory agents, or who were on treatment with calcium channel blocking agents, for indomethicin has been documented to enhance coronary artery vasoconstriction [11], and the calcium channel blocking agents have been documented to blunt the vasoconstrictor response to alpha-adrenergic stimulation [12]. Treatment with beta-adrenergic blocking agents was discontinued for 24 h prior to cardiac catheterization, and long-acting nitrate preparations were held. Following diagnostic cardiac catheterization, a coronary sinus thermodilution pacing catheter was positioned into the coronary sinus by an antecubital vein. The position of the catheter was held constant throughout the subsequent study. Phasic arterial and mean blood pressures were recorded by a femoral artery catheter, arterial and coronary sinus oxygen content measured and arterial and coronary sinus lactate concentrations were measured by an enzymatic spectrophotometric analysis. Measurements of phasic and mean arterial pressure, heart rate, and coronary blood flow, as determined by both coronary sinus thermodilution technique and arterial coronary sinus oxygen content, were made in three states (at rest, during pacing to a subanginal heart rate of 95 ± 5 beats/min to eliminate the influence of change in heart rate on coronary blood flow determinations, and at the same subanginal paced heart rate during the alpha-adrenergic stimulation of the cold pressor test). Such alpha-adrenergic challenge was performed as previously described [5], consisting of immersing the patient's hand

and forearm in ice and water for a minimum of 60 s. Such stimulus is quikly perceived as a noxious, painful stimulus, rather than cold exposure. After initial resting hemodynamics, as well as pacing and cold pressor hemodynamics were obtained, and after pressures returned to baseline, 100 mg of trimazosin, a selective alpha-1 adrenergic blocking agent, was administered intravenously over three minutes. No patient experienced any adverse effect to trimazosin administration. Mean arterial pressure, coronary sinus blood flow, and arterial-coronary sinus O_2 content were obtained at rest, at the same identical subanginal paced heart rate, 5 min and 30 min following trimazosin administration, and once again during the alpha-adrenergic stimulus of cold exposure at the identical heart rate. Arterial and coronary sinus catecholamines were also collected in heparinized syringes through the arterial and coronary sinus catheters during rest, and following administration of trimazosin. No samples were obtained during the cold pressor test, for this is known to enhance myocardial release of catecholamines.

It is interesting to note that in the resting state in supine position, trimazosin administration caused a small but insignificant fall in arterial pressure from 100 ± 15 mmHg to 94 ± 11 mmHg, with minimal decrease in coronary blood from 102 ± 35 ml/min to 91 ± 42 ml/min. Thus, coronary vascular resistance minimally increased (not significantly) from 1.12 ± 0.53 to $1.24 \pm .58$ mmHg/ml/min.

The initial cold pressure test prior to trimazosin administaration, with heart rate maintained constant at 95 ± 5 beats/min, induced a 9% increase in mean arterial pressure, from 100 ± 15 to 109 ± 15 mmHG. This was associated with a concomitant fall in coronary sinus blood flow of 6%, from 102 ± 35 to 97 ± 36 ml/min. Coronary vascular resistance, calculated as the ratio of mean arterial pressure divided by coronary blood flow, increased by 20% from 1.12 ± 0.53 to 1.32 ± 0.68 ($p<0.01$). Trimazosin administration did not significantly alter the hypertensive response to the cold presssor tests, for mean arterial pressure increased by 8% from 94 ± 11 to 102 ± 12 mmHg. However, there was no change in coronary sinus blood flow, and hence, coronary vascular resistance did not significantly increase as during control observations. It might be noted that the product of heart rate times mean arterial pressure, a rough approximation of myocardial oxygen demand, was similar before and after trimazosin administration.

Importantly, there were no significant increases in serum norepinephrine level following trimasozin administration.

The preliminary results of this study indicate that selective alpha-1 adrenergic blockade with trimazosin may attenuate the coronary artery vasoconstriction that is elicited by the alpha-adrenergic stimulus of cold exposure. These findings seem consistent with the animal studies that have reported reduction in coronary vasomotor tone with alpha-1 adrenergic blockade [13]. Alpha-1 adrenergic blockade may have been an advantage over nonselective alpha-adrenergic blocking agents to improve coronary artery blood flow, for selective alpha-1 adrenergic blockade generates vasodilation without further release of catecholamines that may increase myocardial oxygen consumption as noted with nonselective alpha-adrenergic blocking agents.

The results of this study suggest that agents which significantly modulate alpha-1 adrenergic tone may improve coronary artery blood flow in a subgroup of patients with ischemic heart disease and superimposed mild coronary artery vasoconstriction, on exposure to cold. The role of alpha-adrenergic receptors in the pathogenesis of coronary artery spasm in other settings must continue to be questioned. There is little evidence at the present time that such epicardial coronary artery spasm is mediated by localized alpha-adrenergic stimulation [14]. However, a recent small series with coronary artery spasm refractory to conventional medical therapy indicates that selective alpha-adrenergic blockade with prazosin administration may be a very effective therapy [15]. The final place of alpha-1 and alpha-2 adrenergic receptors in patients with coronary artery disease must await further clinical investigations. These changes may be of importance in a subset of patients in whom intense alpha-adrenergic stimulation may result in increased coronary artery vasoconstrictor tone, and adversely influence the balance between myocardial oxygen supply and demand.

References

1. Feigl EO: Sympathetic control of coronary circulation. Circ Res 20:262–271, 1967.
2. Berne RM, DeGeest H, Levy MN: Influence of the cardiac nerves on coronary resistance. Am J Physiol 208:763–769, 1965.
3. Vatner SF, Franklin D, Van Citters RL et al: Effects of carotid sinus nerve stimulation on the coronary circulation of the conscious dog. Cir Res 27:11–21, 1970.
4. Orlick AE, Ricci DR, Alderman EL, Stinson EB, Harrison DC: Effects of alpha-adrenergic blockade upon coronary hemodynamics. J Clin Invest 62:459, 1978.
5. Mudge GH, Grossman W, Mills RM Jr, Lesch M, Braunwald E: Reflex increase in coronary vascular resistance in patients with ischemic heart disease. N Engl J Med 295:1333–1337, 1976.
6. Malacoff RF, Mudge GH Jr, Holman BL, Idoine J, Bifolck Pf: Effect of the cold pressor test on regional myocardial blood flow in patients with coronary artery disease. Am Heart J 106:78–84, 1983.
7. Raizner AE, Chahine RA, Ishimori T: Provocation of coronary artery spasm by the cold pressor test. Hemodynamic, arteriographic and quantitative angiographic observations. Circulation 62:925, 1980.
8. Robertson D, Robertson RM, Nies AS, Oates JA, Friesinger GC: Variant angina pectoris: Investigations of indexes of sympathetic nervous system function. Am J Cardiol 43:1080, 1979.
9. Kern MJ, Ganz P, Horowitz JD, Gaspar J, Barry WH, Lorell BH, Grossman W, Mudge GH Jr: Potentiation of coronary vasoconstriction by beta-adrenergic blockade in patients with coronary artery disease. Circulation 67:1178–1185, 1983.
10. Kern M, Horowitz JD, Ganz P, Gaspar J, Colucci WS, Lorell B, Barry WH, Mudge GH: Selective alpha-1 adrenergic mediated coronary vasoconstriction in patients with coronary artery disease (in press).
11. Friedman PL, Brown EJ Jr, Gunther S, Alexander RW, Barry WH, Mudge GH Jr, Grossman W:

Coronary vasoconstriction effect of indomethacin in patients with coronary artery disease. N Engl J Med 305:1171–1175, 1981.

12. Gunther S, Muller JE, Mudge GH, Grossman W: Therapy of coronary vasoconstriction in patients with coronary artery disease. Am J Cardiol 47:157–162, 1981.

13. Macho P, Hintze TH, Vatner SF: Effects of alpha-adrenergic receptor blockade on coronary circulation in conscious dogs. Am J Physiol 243:H94–H98, 1982.

14. Chierchia S. The role of alpha-adrenergic receptors in the pathogenesis of coronary spasm. Clin Cardiol 6:496–500, 1983.

15. Tzivoni D, Keren A, Benhorin Jesaia, Gottlieb S, Atlas D, Stern S: Prazosin therapy for refractory variant angina. Am Heart J 105:262–264, 1983.

Discussion

Dr. McGregor: What was the myocardial oxygen consumption after alpha-blockade?

Dr. Mudge: In our protocol it did not change, but we only measured $AV\text{-}O_2$-differences in a small number of patients.

Dr. Serruys: Stimulated by your work several groups in Europe have tried to reproduce the study. It was quite difficult to reduce coronary blood flow during the cold pressor test. It seems that the major difference between the studies is that you have paced your patients. My question is: What was the anginal threshold for pacing induced angina in these patients, in other words, was your pacing rate during cold pressor test submaximal?

Dr Mudge: That is a very important question. In those patients with a very low anginal threshold, we can see increases in coronary vascular resistance during the cold pressor test of about 50%. On the other hand, in those patients with the similar same angiographycally documented coronary artery stenoses but a much higher anginal threshold during pacing, we have not seen as significant a change in coronary vascular resistance.

I think the important point I would like to emphasize is that we have not looked especially for a drop in blood flow, although we have seen that.

Dr. McGregor: In normal individuals or in patients who are very well below the anginal threshold, there is an autoregulatory capacity which will compensate for any upstream vasoconstriction. And I wonder if you have ever considered getting around that by first abolishing autoregulatory capacity with a drug like persantine? Williams and Most did something like that using adenosine to abolish autoregulation. Thereafter manipulation of the upstream resistance by a vasopressor could be shown to reduce flow. This could not be shown while autoregulation was intact.

Dr. Mudge: We have not looked at the autoregulatory reserve.

Dr. Bassenge: During electrical stimulation of the cardiac sympathetic nerves under β-blockade we got a much stronger decline in coronary flow or a much stronger increase in coronary resistance by application of the selective alpha$_2$-

blocking agent Rauwolscine. So at least in the canine coronary bed the signifi-cance of alpha$_2$ coronary vasoconstriction is probably more pronounced.

Dr. Vatner: I would like to make a couple of suggestions: (1) Try a non-selective vasodilator to make sure that it is not the vasodilating action of Trimazosin which is blocking the effects. (2) If you have the oportunity to deliver your blocker directly into the coronary circulation and leaving the systemic response intact, you could differentiate wheter all these effects are the result of an increased pressure and calculated coronary vascular resistance or whether they are directley mediated.

Dr. Mudge: These studies are actually on-going. We are using at the moment, a streptokinase catheter placed across a non-spastic artherosclerotic lesion, there-by getting the distal perfusion pressure and recording central aortic pressure. We are then performing distal coronary injections of either β-blocking agents or calcium channel blockers, and measuring changes of coronary vascular resistance in proximal conductance and distal resistance vessels.

Dr. Vatner: It would be very interesting to inject alpha blockers and see whether you get the same changes in coronary resistance .

Dr. McGregor: In this way you also would avoid the changes in collateral flow, which must be a confusing factor.

9. The effect of cardioselective beta blockade by metoprolol on the coronary vascular tone under endogenous catecholamine stimulation

C.W. HAMM, A. DEPPE, W. BLEIFELD & W. KUPPER

Introduction

The administration of beta-adrenergic antagonists to patients with stable or unstable angina pectoris is a well-established therapeutic regime [2]. The effectiveness of these compounds has been related to the reduction in oxygen demand due to the attenuated myocardial response to sympathetic stimuli [2]. However, in patients with variant angina there has been some concern that beta-blockade promotes coronary artery spasm [10]. Recent reports revealed that critical changes in the tone of large, epicardial coronary arteries may occur despite any history typical for vasotonic angina [6]. Moreover, Kern et al. [4] demonstrated recently that the non-selective, beta antagonist propranolol potentiates the increase in coronary vascular resistance due to increased sympathetic outflow by means of the cold pressor test. The authors proposed to relate this effect to the unmasked alpha-adrenergic vasomotor tone. Based on these observations, the present study was designed to investigate whether cardioselective beta-blockade by metoprolol is associated with unfavorable effects on coronary vascular resistance and on the tone of large coronary arteries in response to endogenous catecholamine liberation.

Patients and methods

The study group consisted of ten patients (all male, 47 ± 6 years) undergoing cardiac catheterization for a chest pain syndrome not typical for variant angina. After informed consent was obtained all medication except short acting nitrates was discontinued at least 24 h prior to the study. Coronary arteriography revealed a single vessel disease with nearly concentric stenoses between 50 and 80% in diameter in two patients, a double vessel disease in three patients and only vessel wall irregularities in the remaining five patients. The left ventricular ejection fraction was in all cases within the normal range of our laboratory (>50%). At least 15 min after completion of the diagnostic procedure, a No 7 F thermodilution coronary sinus catheter (Wilton Webster, Altadena, Ca, USA) was introduced

Kupper, W. (ed.), Coronary tone in ischemic heart disease. ISBN 0-89838-646-2.

96

into an antecubital vein and advanced under fluoroscopic guidance to the mid-coronary sinus. The stable position of the coronary sinus catheter was confirmed repeatedly by fluoroscopy and injection of contrast medium. Coronary sinus blood flow was measured as described by Ganz [3] at an injection rate of 36 ml/min of 5% glucose.

Pulmonary pressures were measured with a No. 7 ballon-tipped catheter inserted through a femoral vein. Aortic pressures were monitored via the left Judkins catheter continously with a 3-lead electrocardiogram on an Electronics for Medicine VR 12 recorder (Diefenbach, Frankfurt/Main, FRG).

Arterial and coronary venous blood samples were obtained simultaneously and analyzed for oxygen and lactate. Serum lactate was determined by standard biochemical methods [1], with the restraints of lactate measurements as pointed out previously [5]. Oxygen content was measured by an electrochemical method (Lex-O_2-Con, Lexington Instruments, Lenxington, TN, USA).

Coronary angiograms of the left coronary artery were obtained in the same RAO 30° position throughout the study. Diameters of the left anterior and circumflex coronary artery were determined by means of a calibre at 15 times magnification. For the analysis it was differentiated between normal and stenotic (>50% mean diameter reduction) segments, as well as segments with vessel wall irregularities. The results of two independent and experienced observers were corrected for magnification by using the circumference of the catheter as standard.

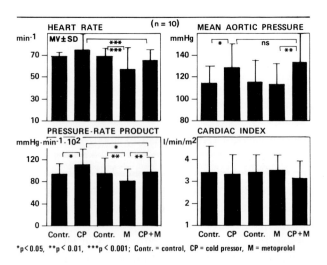

Figure 1. Heart rate, mean aortic pressure, rate product and cardiac index in response to the cold pressor test before and after 5 mg metoprolol.

Data analysis

Cardiac output was calculated according to Fick. Cardiac index was determined by cardiac output divided by the surface area ($l/min/m^2$). The heart rate-blood pressure double product was obtained by systolic aortic pressure × heart rate (mmHg/min). The transmyocardial lactate extraction rate (LE) was calculated as:

$$LE\ (\%) = \frac{(Lactate)_{art} - (Lactate)_{cor-ven}}{(Lactate)_{art}} \times 100,$$

where $(lactate)_{art}$ is the arterial lactate concentration and $(lactate)_{cor-ven}$ is the concentration in the coronary sinus. Myocardial oxygen consumption (MVO_2) was calculated by the equation MVO_2 (ml/min) = coronary sinus blood flow × ($O_2art - O_2cor-ven$).

Protocol

First all hemodynamic and metabolic baseline measurements were obtained and baseline angiography was performed. Then the patient's hand and forearm were immersed in ice water and the patient was asked to stir the water for 60 sec. Occurence of chest pain or a rise in systolic blood pressure by more than 30 mmHg were considered as criteria of premature termination. All recordings were taken within the last 15 sec of the cold pressor rest and angiography was performed when the patient lifted his hand out of the water. After at least 20 min, when baseline values were reestablished, 5 mg of metoprolol (Astra Chemicals, Wedel/Holstein, FRG) was given intravenously over a period of 5 min. There is valid evidence that at this dose effective beta-blockade is achieved. After another 5 min all measurements were repeated and the second cold pressor test was carried out with all parameters obtained. The reproducibility of the cold pressor test was shown earlier.

Statistical analysis

Results are expressed as mean ± SD, and P values were calculated by the appropriate Student's t-test and $p < 0.05$ was considered significant.

Results

The hemodynamic and metabolic response to the cold pressor test and to meto-

98

prolol was very similar in patients with or without coronary artery obstructions. For this reason the results have been compiled in the following manner.

1. Hemodynamic results. In response to the cold pressor test, heart rate increased from 70 ± 5/min to 74 ± 15 (n.s.) and aortic pressure from 132 ± 21 to 148 ± 28 (p<0.05). The rate pressure product, as an index of myocardial oxygen demand, was augmented from 93 ± 20 mmHg/min $\times 10^2$ to 110 ± 29 mmHg/min $\times 10^{-2}$ (Figure 1). The parameters returned to baseline values and the application of metoprolol was followed by the well-known decrease in heart rate (from 69 ± 7 to 57 ± 20, p<0.001) and rate pressure product (94 ± 29 $81 + 22$, p<0.01). The mean aortic pressure did not change significantly. In the ensuing cold pressor test

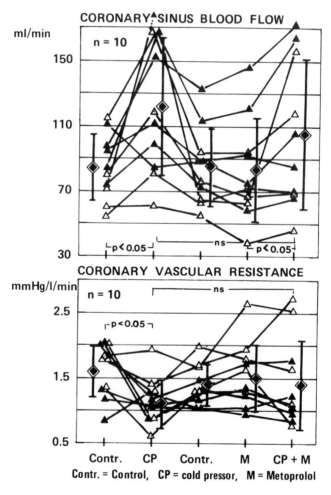

Figure 2. Coronary sinus blood flow and coronary vascular resistance in response to the cold pressor test before and after 5 mg metoprolol

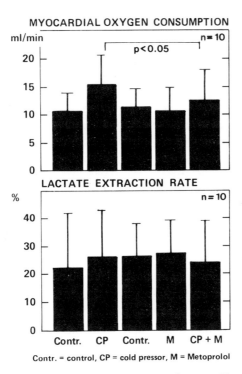

MYOCARDIAL OXYGEN CONSUMPTION

LACTATE EXTRACTION RATE

Contr. = control, CP = cold pressor, M = Metoprolol

*Figure 3.*Myocardial oxygen consumption and lactate extraction rate. There was no production of lactate in any patient during the study.

heart rate (65 ± 11/min, $p<0.001$) and rate-pressure product (97 ± 29, $p<0.05$) increased less compared with the cold pressor test before beta-blockade (Figure 1). The cardiac index exhibited no significant change throughout the study.

Parallel to the rate- pressure product, coronary sinus blood flow increased in response to the cold pressor test from 84 ± 20 ml/min to 122 ± 42 ml/min ($p<0.05$) and in the presence of metoprolol from 83 ± 32 ml/min to 105 ± 46 ml/min ($p<0.05$) The rise after metoprolol was not as pronounced as under control conditions; however, this did not reach the level of significance (Figure 2). Due to the small increase in aortic pressure related to the rise in coronary sinus blood flow, coronary vascular resistance decreased during the cold pressor test from 1.6 ± 0.40 to 1.1 ± 0.37 mmHg/min ($p<0.05$), but not significantly after metoprolol (1.41 ± 0.69) (Figure 2).

2. Metabolic results. The enhanced oxygen demand as indicated by the elevated pressure-rate product was followed by increased oxygen uptake during the cold pressor test from 11.3 ± 3.1 ml/min to 15.2 ± 6.1. ml/min. Accordingly, the oxygen consumption in the presence of metoprolol was less (8.8 ± 2.9 ml/min, $p<0.05$)

under this stimulation (Figure 3). In all cases the oxygen demand was sufficiently met by the oxygen supply as concluded from the lactate extraction rate (Figure 3). Lactate production did not occur in any of the cases.

3. Magnification angiography. The metabolic observation that oxygen supply was not critically reduced was supported by the evaluation of the coronary artery diameters. There was a general trend to a reduction in diameter in the cold pressor test; however, even under metroprolol no higher degree obstruction could be observed in normal vessels or vessels with minor wall irregularities (Figure 4).

The diameters of the coronary artery stenoses in the five patients with relevant coronary artery disease were analyzed separately. As depicted in Table 1, there was no directed trend, and no harmful effect on the coronary artery stenoses diameter could be detected.

Discussion

The angiographic, metabolic and hemodynamic results of the present study demonstrate that in patients without a history of variant angina, cardioselective,

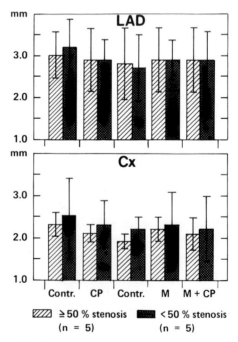

Figure 4. Quantitative magnification angiography of normal segments in the left anterior descending and circumflex artery.

Table 1. Quantitative magnification angiography of stenotic lesions (mm diameter). No directed change was apparent after metoprolol.

	Control		Cold pressor		Metoprolol		Metoprolol + Cold Pressor	
	LAD	Cx	LAD	Cx	LAD	Cx	LAD	Cx
1	1.9	–	1.9	–	1.8	–	1.8	–
2	–	1.1	–	1.0–		1.1	–	1.0
3	–	1.4	–	1.8	–	1.4	–	1.6
4	1.1	1.5	1.2	1.4	1.2	1.5	1.3	1.4
5	1.4	2.1	1.3	1.4	1 .4	1.7	1.1	1.6

beta-adrenergic antagonism by metoprolol is not associated with detrimental side-effects on the coronary vascular tone. This has been shown at rest and during endogenous catecholamine liberation by means of the cold pressor test. These findings are therefore in agreement with the broad clinical experience that beta-blockade is an effective and safe therapy in patients with coronary heart disease. The design of our study was tailored to the typical patient with coronary heart disease, who receives beta-blocking medication and who is exposed to sympathetic stress as mimiced in our case by exposure to cold. We investigated the effect of metoprolol on the large conductance vessels by magnification angiography as well as on the resistance vessels by calculation of the coronary vascular resistance.

In patients with variant angina it has been reported [10] that beta-blockade may aggravate indirect signs of myocardial ischemia, e.g. ECG-ST-segment depression and duration of anginal attacks. There is no further evidence whether this unfavorable effect is related to changes in tone of large coronary arteries or of resistance vessels. For large coronary arteries it has been proposed that beta-blockade may induce vasoconstriction due to the predominance of alpha-unopposed adrenergic tone [4] or as a result of reduced myocardial oxygen demand [9]. Vatner and Hintze [12] demonstrated that the constriction in large coronary arteries appears to be mainly mediated by the concomitant metabolic effects of beta-blockade. However, substantial vasoconstriction could only be observed in the presence of elevated beta-1-adrenergic tone and/or metabolic vasodilation, but our investigation was not performed in a state of exhausted vasodilatory reserve. Therefore we probably missed small changes in coronary artery tone which might have occured. In addition the resolution of magnification angiography is certainly associated with remarkable limitations compared with experimental set ups.

As opposed to the patients Kern et al. [4] investigated we did not find a rise in coronary vascular resistance induced by the cold pressor test, even in the presence of metoprolol. Two explanations can be put forward to explain this discrepancy. First, our patients were not paced to subanginal heart rates; therefore their autoregulatory reserve was not exhausted and they could respond to the stress with elevated blood flow. Secondly, Kern and co-workers achieved beta-block-ade with the non-selective compound propranolol. Preliminary results indicate [6] that the evaluation in coronary vascular resistance may be associated with non-selective beta-blockade but not with selective by metoprolol. However, the clinical relevance of these observations remains limited, since thus far no signs of myocardial ischemia have been detected and related to beta-blockade in any patient.

References

1. Bergmeyer HM: Methoden der enzymatischen Analyse II. Verlag Chemie, Weinheim, 1974.
2. Frishman W, Silverman R: Clinical pharmacalology of the new beta-adrenergic blocking drugs. Part II: Physiologic and metabolic effects. Am Heart J 97:797–807, 1979.
3. Ganz W, Tamura K, Marcus HS, Donoso R, Yoshida S, Swan HJC: Measurement of coronary sinus blood flow by continuous thermodilution in man. Circulation 44:181–195, 1971.
4. Kern MJ, Ganz P, John D, Horowitz JG, Barry WH, Lorell BH, Grossman W, Mudge GH: Potentiation of coronary vasoconstriction by beta-adrenergic blockade in patients with coronary artery disease. Circulation 67:1178–1185, 1983.
5. Kupper W, Bleifeld W: Measurement of regional and global coronary sinus blood flow with the continuous thermodilution technique. II. Clinical studies in patients with coronary heart disease. Z Kardiol 70:116–123, 1981.
6. Kupper W, Hamm CW, Gublass U, Bleifeld W: Induction of coronary artery spasm in patients without history of variant angina by cold pressor or ergonovine testing. Eur Heart J 4 (suppl E):45, 1983.
7. Kupper W, Schütt M, Hamm CW, Kuck KH, Hanrath P, Bleifeld W: Haemodynamic and cardiac metabolis effects of the new β-agonist prenaterol in patients with cardiac failure. Eur Heart J 4:573–583, 1983.
8. Kupper W, Hamm CW, Bleifeld W: Effect of non-selective and selective β-adrenergic blockade on coronary artery tone. Circulation 68:II–73, 1983.
9. Parratt JR: Myocardial metabolic activity as a determinant of coronary vessel tone. In: Kalmer S (ed) The coronary artery. Croom Helm, London pp 309–339, 1982.
10. Robertson RM, Wood AJJ, Vaughn WK, Robertson D: Exacerbation of vasotonic angina pectoris by propranolol. Circulation 65:281–285, 1982.
11. Vatner SF, Hintze TH, Macho P: Regulation of large coronary arteries by β-adrenergic mecha-nisms in the conscious dog. Circ Res 51:56–66, 1982.
12. Vatner SF, Hintze TH: Mechanism of constriction of large coronary arteries by β-adrenergic receptor blockade. Circ Res 53:389–400, 1983.

Discussion

Dr. Vatner: I have no objections to any of your results. I think you found that the beta-blocker did not have any significant effects and there was no difference in response to the cold pressor test. But this is not the same thing as studying a patient with a high level of sympathetic tone and then giving your beta-blockers in the presence of the high level of sympathetic tone.

What we did in a series of animal experiments was to give atenelol in the presence of high catecholamine levels. We found a very dramatic reduction in coronary artery dimensions. But if we gave the beta-blocker in the absence of high catecholamine levels, we saw only very small reductions in coronary artery diameters. I could understand how clinical techniques would not be able to discern such small changes.

Dr. Hamm: Certainly the limitations of magnification angiography do not allow to detect such small changes as you observed in your fine animal experiments. The object of our study was, however, to see, whether we could find localized spasms of coronary arteries more frequently in the presence of beta-blockade. We and others have demonstrated earlier that such spasms do occur during the cold pressor test and can be detected by magnification angiography. Our protocol was designed for the typical patient, treated with beta-blockers, who is exposed to adrenergic stress. The situation that someone receives acutely only beta-blockers in the presence of high levels of catecholamines appears in the clinical setting rather rare and was therefore not the matter of investigation of this study.

Dr. Mudge: I think this is an important observation, because your conclusions may be important for about 95% of our coronary patients. However, there are some rare reports that beta-adrenoceptor blockade makes coronary spasm worse. We have completed a study where we tried to exhaust vasodilatory reserve of the patients by rapid atrial pacing up to heart rate of approximately 100/min. We then gave 0.1 mg/kg propranolol, and what we found is a substantial increase in coronary vascular resistance in some patients.

Dr. Hamm: Thank you for pointing out the basic difference in the protocol between your study and ours. However, the discrepancy we found in coronary vascular resistance may be also due–in part–to the two different drugs.

Dr. Bassenge: Robertson (Circulation 1982) and Bertrand (Am. J. Cardiol. 1983) reported a higher incidence of coronary spasm in patients after administration of beta-blocking agents. I think these were selected patients with proven Prinzmetal angina, whereas in your study you have just a mixture containing mainly fixed arteriosclerotic stenosis which may be very little influenced by changes in sympathetic tone.

Dr. Hamm: I think that there is ample evidence now that coronary arteries with arteriosclerotic lesions underly important changes in tone (Gould 1980, Rafflenbeul 1982). Fixed stenoses appear to be rather the exception. To our observation significant changes in coronary artery tone occur even predominantly in segments with wall irregularities.

Dr. Mueller: I want to emphasize that of Dr. Bassenge, Roberts et al. did not show an increased *incidence*, but an increased *duration* of variant aninal attacks.

104

Dr. Bassenge: An increased duration and severity, they measured it in terms of ST-segment depression.

Dr. Chierchia: We are all aware of this study but it seems, we have forgotten another study by Guazzi and co workers (1976) who gave large doses of practolol and propranolol to patients with diagnosed Prinzmetal angina. The vast maiorty of the patients responded to this treatment.

Dr. Serruys: But the dose was 1000 mg, and with this dose you have some kind of calcium blocking effects.

Dr. Chierchia: The effect was certainly not related to the sympathetic activity blocking effect of drug.

Dr. Serruys: Two years ago we did a similar kind of study combining blood flow measurements with thermodilution and quantitative coronary angiography and got exactly the same results. Even if we included six patients with unstable angina which reported an increase of their frequency of anginal attacks during cold exposure during their daily activities, we were unable to show any significant change in the diameter of the coronary system.

10. Alpha-adrenergic receptors and coronary vasospasm

S. CHIERCHIA

Introduction

Stimulation of coronary alpha-adrenergic receptors has been repeatedly impli-
cated as a mechanism potentially responsible for coronary spasm. This hypothesis
is certainly supported by the experimental observation that coronary arteries are
densely innervated with sympathetic fibres and that reflex and pharmacological
stimulation of alpha-adrenergic receptors produces vasoconstriction. However,
the clinical evidence to support the hypothesis is only based on isolated and rather
anecdotal observations reporting that spasm can be precipitated by alpha-adrenergic stimulation and prevental or reserved by alpha-blockade.

This paper will briefly summarise the results of experimental and human
studies investigating the response of the coronary vasculature to sympathetic
stimulation and present the current evidence supporting or disproving the role of
alpha receptors in the initiation of coronary artery spasm.

Experimental observations

All coronaries, down to the smallest arterioles, have extensive adrenergic innervation [1]. Histochemical studies have shown a preponderance of alpha receptors
in the larger epicardial vessels, while beta receptors predominate in small arteries
[1]. In various animal preparations, stimulation of cardiac sympathetic nerves
invariably causes the coronary blood flow to increase [2]. However, a reduction in
flow is observed if the chronotropic and inotropic effects of adrenergic stimulation are prevented by beta blockade and activation of alpha receptors is unmasked [2]. Coronary vasoconstriction mediated by stimulation of alpha receptors has also been obtained with stimulation of the posterior hypothalumus [3]
with baroreceptor hypotension after beta blockade [4].

A tonic alpha-adrenergic coronary vasoconstrictor activity has been shown in
the dog both at rest and during exercise; this can be reflexly reduced by carotid
sinus nerve stimulation or phentolamine [5, 6]; Similar findings have been obtained in man by Orlick et al. [7]; these authors measured coronary blood flow by

Kupper, W. (ed.), Coronary tone in ischemic heart disease. ISBN 0-89838-646-2.
© *1984, Martinus Nijhoff Publishers, Boston/The Hague/Dordrecht/Lancaster. Printed in the Netherlands.*

thermodilution and found evidence for a basal coronary constrictor tone which was reduced by phentolamine and absent in patients with transplanted, denervated hearts.

Injection of noradrenaline into vein grafts at coronary bypass surgery resulted in a large, transient reduction of coronary flow, due to activation of alpha-adrenergic receptors [8]. The same receptors probably mediate the reduction in coronary blood flow observed in patients with coronary artery disease during the cold pressor test [9]. Coronary arteriography during 'cold pressor' reveals only minimal changes in the diameter of epicardial arteries [10]; the observed changes in coronary vascular resistance and flow are thus likely to be consequent to constriction of the small resistance vessels which are not visualised at angiography.

Alpha-receptors mediated constriction of large epicardial arteries has been convincingly demonstrated in vitro and vivo. In 1912 Barbour obtained human coronary arteries soon after death and produced strong constrictions after adding adrenaline to the organ bath [11]. Kountz using a similar technique showed that low concentrations of adrenaline produced contraction, while higher concentrations caused relaxation [12]. More recently, Ginsburg et al. [13] studied the effects of various vasoactive drugs on fresh human arteries from heart transplant recipients and found that their basal tone was not affected by alpha or beta blockade. The arteries responed to alpha and beta stimulation, but the magnitude of alpha constriction was comparatively small when compared to beta dilation.

Constriction of large epicardial arteries in response to intravenous methoxamine, a powerful alpha-adrenergic agonist, has been described in concious, chronically instrumented dogs [14]. The reduction in coronary diameter occured in the presence of a marked increase of aortic pressure and hence of coronary distending pressure; however, coronary blood flow was not apparently affected. Minor reductions in coronary diameter have also been reported in man, at coronary arteriography, during handgrip and after administration of epinephrine following beta blockade [15]. In patients with 'variant' angina, constriction of stenosed coronary segments after epinephrine appeared greater than in patients with stenoses of similar severity and 'noncardiac' chest pain [15].

Alpha-adrenergic receptors and 'variant' angina

In 1974 Yasue et al. gathered three patients with variant angina in whom transient ST-segment elevation could be provoked by the parasympathomimetic agent methacholine, and by epinephrine (2 patients). Methacholine was believed to induce spasm by releasing norepinephrine from postganglionic sympathetic nerve endings; the fact that the drug predominantly acts on muscarinic cholinergic receptors, and has little, if any, nicotinic effects, was disregarded. In all patients symptoms were prevented by atropine and apparently exacerbated by propranolol. Alpha blockade with phenoxybenzamine appeared to prevent, in one patient, the occurence of spontaneous episodes of vasospastic angina [16]. Two years later the same group published a report on three other patients in whom coronary spasm could be consistently reproduced by the combined administration of oral propranolol and subcutaneous adrenaline. Again, propranolol appeared to make symptoms worse. The authors concluded that 'Prinzmetal variant angina is caused by severe spasm of a large coronary artery mediated by alpha-adrenergic receptors' [17].

Further evidence to support this hypothesis came from Ricci et al. who noted prolongation of the corrected QT interval before the onset of ST-segment elevation and spasm either occuring spontaneously or induced by ergonovine maleate. QT prolongation was not observed in a group of control patients who did not respond to ergonovine. The authors proposed that QT prolongation and the spasm which followed were the result of asymmetrical stellate ganglion activity and transient alpha-adrenergic stimulation. Spasm was reserved at angiography by intravenous phentolamine in eight patients and prevented in four for a period of 2–3 months follow-up with phenoxybenzamine [18].

Stimulation of coronary alpha-adrenergic receptors has also been proposed to be responsible for exercise-induced spasm. The hypothesis was first put forward by Levene and Freeman, who published the earliest specific report on coronary spasm during exercise. They described a patient with angina at rest and on exercise, on whom spontaneous coronary spasm, relieved by phentolamine, occured at angiography. Alpha blockade with phenoxybenzamine prevented exercise-induced ST elevation and the authors concluded that alpha-mediated coronary spasm was the cause of ischaemia during exercise [19]. Yasue et al. found phentolamine effective in preventing exercise coronary spasm in 26 patients while propanolol was ineffective.

Other physical maneuvres known to increase the sympathetic activity to the heart, such as the cold pressor test, have also been occasionally reported to precipitate coronary spasm [10]. In our hands the cold pressor test is as much as ten times less sensitive than ergonovine in provoking spasm, and is usually effective only in highly susceptible patients with a high daily frequency of spontaneous episodes of vasospastic ischaemia. Other authors report a similar experience [19].

The first study challenging the hypothesis of alpha-receptor mediated coronary spasm was published by Robertson et al. who performed, in three patients with frequent episodes of spasm and only minor coronary lesions, a battery of tests to evaluate sympathetic function [20]. No apparent resting abnormalities were found, and when compared to a group of normal controls, no differences were evident. Plasma catecholamine levels were not increased during control nor at the onset of the attacks, and in one patient there was no change in forearm venous compliance (an index of alpha-adrenergic tone) just before an ischaemic episode. In another study the same group obtained arterial and coronary sinus blood

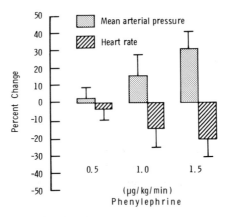

Figure 1. Haemodynamic response to three increasing doses of phenylephrine. Although in all patients the drug induced a dose-dependent increase in mean arterial pressure and a reflex decrease in heart rate, in no instances did it produce coronary spasm.

samples to measure catecholamine levels during control, at the beginning and in the late phase of episodes of ischaemia due to coronary spasm. No significant differences between control and beginning of ischaemia could be found although both arterial and coronary sinus catecholamines increased in the late phase of the episodes. The authors concluded that increased sympathetic activity to the heart was likely to be a consequence of ischaemia rather than the cause of spasm [21]. The beneficial effects of atropine, reported by Yasue in patients with variant angina, could not be confirmed by other studies [22, 23].

In 15 patients with variant angina high-dose propranolol and practolol (up to 800 and 2000 mg respectively) were reported by Guazzi et al. to be highly effective in preventing episodes of ischaemia [24]. Treatment with beta blockers fully abolished the attacks in about two-thirds of the patients; some patients unresponsive to one beta blocker did not respond to the other. The dose of the drug was titrated to individual response with a large patient-to-patient variability and was always higher than that required to prevent isoprenaline-induced ta-chycardia; this suggests that mechanisms other than beta blockade accounted for the therapeutic effect. No patients showed exacerbation of symptoms and/or ischaemia while on beta blockers.

In a group of 14 consecutive patients with variant angina, we recently per-formed a systematic study aimed at investigation the role of alpha receptors in the initiation of coronary artery spasm [25]. Patients underwent serial provocative testing during continuous ECG, arterial pressure and left ventricular function monitoring. With ergonovine, all patients exhibited pain and/or transient ST-seg-ment elevation, accompanied by severe impairment of left ventricular function. Stepwise infusion of phenylephrine or noradrenaline after beta blockade consistently produced a marked, dose-dependent increase in blood pressure accompanied by a reflex decrease in heart rate (Figure 1); in no instance did the administration of these drugs result in ECG or left ventricular function changes suggestive of spasm or ischaemia.

Cold pressor test produced ST-segment elevation and spasm only in one patient who had a very high daily incidence of spontaneous ischaemic episodes, as documented by continuous Holter monitoring. The reproducibility of the response to the cold pressor was checked in this patient on three separate occasions and proved to be variable; the test was either negative or positive with ST-segment elevation or depression on the same electrocardiographic leads.

Beat-by beat, computerised measurement of heart rate and corrected QT interval showed no significant increase in these parameters in the period preceding the onset of transient ST-segment changes recorded during continuous 24-h ambulatory ECG monitoring [25] (Figure 2). Analysis of the circadian distribution of episodes of vasospastic ischeamia confirmed a prevalence of nocturnal episodes with a peak in the early morning hours when sympathetic activity is known to be at its lowest level [25] (Figure 3).

In five patients, continuous intravenous infusion of phentolamine did not affect the frequency of episodes of vasospastic ischaemia when compared to placebo [25] (Figure 4). Although we cannot rule out catecholamine overflow due to alpha$_2$-presynaptic-receptor blockade by phentolamine, similar negative results have been reported in a recent study in which prazosin, a selective alpha$_1$ antagonist, was given to six patients with variant angina [26].

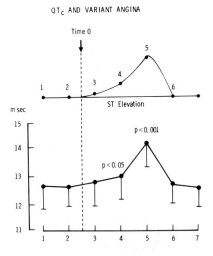

Figure 2. Behaviour of the corrected Q-T interval (mean + SD calculated on all episodes) during control (1, 2), ischaemia (3, 4, 5) and recovery (6, 7). Q-T interval prolongation is observed during but not before ST segment elevation.

110

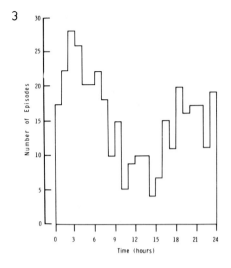

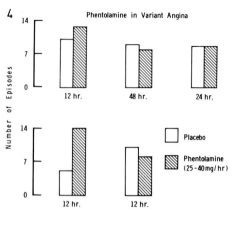

Figure 3. Diurnal distribution of episodes of ischaemia showing a peak incidence in the early morning hours, when the sympathetic tone is at its lowest level.

Figure 4. Effect of intravenous phentolamine (as compared to placebo) on episodes of vasospastic myocardial ischaemia in five patients with variant angina.

Conclusions

The evidence summarised in this review indicates that alpha-receptor mediated spasm remains an attractive, yet unproven, pathophysiological hypotheses, based more on anecdotal reports than on extensive, systematic studies.

The result of our and other author's studies seem to rule out the possibility that a generalised increase in the sympathetic outflow to the heart can initiate coronary spasm, although localised alpha-adrenergic stimulation of epicardial arteries cannot be excluded.

References

1. King MP, Angelalsos ET, Uzgiris I: Innervation of the coronaries (abstract). Fed Proc 30:613, 1971.
2. Feigl EO: Sympathetic control of coronary circulation. Circ Res 20:262, 1967.
3. Alanis J, Lopes E, Rosas O: Changes in dog's coronary circulation by hypothalamic stimulation. Arch Inst Cardiol Mex 22:743, 1962.
4. Hacket JG, Abboud FM, Mark AL. Schmid PG, Heistad DD: Coronary vascular responses to stimulation of chemoreceptors and baroreceptor. Circ Res 31:8, 1972.
5. Murray PA, Vatner SF: Alpha-receptor attenuation of the coronary vascular response to severe, spontaneous exercise in the conscious dog. Circ Res 45:654, 1979.
6. Vatner SF. Franklin D, Van Citters RL: Effects of carotid sinus nerve stimulation on the coronary circulation of the conscious dog. Circ Res 27:11, 1970.

7. Orlick AE, Ricci DR, Alderman EL, Stinson EB, Harrison DC: Effects of alpha-adrenergic blockade upon coronary haemodynamics. J Clin Invest 62:459, 1978.
8. Greenfield JC, Rembert JC, Young JG Jr, Oldham NH Jr, Alexander JA, Sabiston DC: Studies of blood flow in aorta to coronary venous bypass grafts in man. J Clin Invest 51:2724, 1972.
9. Mudge GH, Grossman W, Mills RM, Lesch M, Braunwald E: Reflex increase in coronary vascular resistance in patients with ischaemic heart disease. N. Engl J Med 295:1333, 1976.
10. Raizner AE, Chachine RA, Ishimori T: Provocation of coronary artery spasm by the cold pressor test. Haemodynamic, arteriographic and quantitative angiographic observations. Circularion 62:925, 1980.
11. Barbour HG: The constricting influence of adrenalin upon the human in coronary arteries. J Exp Med 15:404, 1912.
12. Kountz WB: Studies in the coronary arteries of the human heart. J Pharmacol Exp Ther 45:65, 1932.
13. Ginsburg R, Bristow ME, Harrison DC, Stinson EB: Studies with isolated human coronary arteries: Some general observations, potential mediators of spasm, role of calcium antagonists. Chest 78 (suppl):180, 1980.
14. Vatner SF, Pagani P, Manders WT, Pasipoularides F: Alpha-adrenergic control of large coronary arterial resistance and elastic stiffness in the conscious dog. In:Les Alphabloquants. Masson, Paris, 1981, pp 167–178.
15. Brown BG, Bolson E, Frimer M, Dodge HT: Angiographic distinction between variant angina and non-vasospastic chest pain (abstract). Circulation 57/58 (suppl II):II–122, 1978.
16. Yasue H, Touyama M, Shimamoto M, Kato H, Tanaka S, Akiyama F: Role of autonomic nervous system in the pathogenesis of Prinzmetal's variant form of angina. Circulation 50:534, 1974.
17. Yasue H, Touyama M, Kato H, Tanaka S, Akiyama F:Prinzmetal's variant form of angina as a manifestation of alpha-adrenergic receptor-mediated coronary artery spasm: documentation by coronary arteriography. Am Heart J 91:148, 1976.
18. Ricci DR, Orlick AE, Cipriano PR, Guthaner DF, Harrison DC: Altered adrenergic activity in coronary arterial spasm: Insight into mechanism based on study of coronary haemodynamics and the electrocardiogram. Am J Cardiol 43:1073, 1979.
19. Waters DJ, Szlachcic J, Bonan R, Miller DD, Franz D, Theroux P: Comparative sensitivity of exercise, cold pressor and ergonovine testing in provoking attacks of variant angina in patients with active disease. Circulation 67:310, 1983.
20. Robertson D, Robertson RM, Nies AS, Oates JA, Friesinger GC: Variant angina pectoris: investigation of indices of sympathetic nervous system function. Am J Cardiol 43:1080, 1979.
21. Robertson RM, Bernard YD, Robertson D: Coronary sinus and arterial catecholamines during coronary spasm (abstract). Circulation 64:245, 1981.
22. Berman ND, McLaughlin PR, Huckell VF, Mahon WA, Morch JE, Adelman AG: Prinzmetal's angina with coronary artery spasm: Angiographic, pharmacologic, metabolic and radionuclide perfusion studies. Am J Med 60:727, 1976.
23. Maseri A, Severi S, Chierchia S, Parodi O, Biagini A: Characteristics, incidence and pathogenetic mechanisms of 'primary' angina at rest. In: Maseri A, Klassen GA, Lesch M (eds). Primary and Secondary Angina Pectoris. Grune and Stratton, New York, 1978, p 265.
24. Guazzi M, Fiorentini C, Polese A, Magnini F, Olivari MT: Use of beta-receptor antagonists in spontaneous angina pectoris. In: Maseri S, Klassen GA, Lesch M (eds). Primary and Secondary Angina Pectoris. Grune and Stratton, New York, 1978.
25. Chierchia S, Davies G, Berkenboom G, Crea F, Crean P, Maseri A: Alpha-adrenergic receptors and coronary spasm: an elusive link. Circulation 69 (in press).
26. Winniford MD, Filipchuck N, Hollis D: Alpha-adrenergic blockade for variant angina: a long term, double-blind, randomised trial. Circulation 67:1185, 1983.

112

Discussion

Dr. McGregor: You have shown us the frequency of anginal attacks in a series of patients with Prinzmetal angina as well as some with classical unstable angina. One would expect a lower exercise threshold in the patients with unstable angina. Did you carry out your alpha stimulating – or blocking manoeuvres also in the group with unstable angina, because many people would expect in this group that the alpha-tone could play a major role.

Dr. Chierchia: No, we have not tried, but I agree that this is a very important point.

Dr. Bleifeld: You showed that frequency of anginal attacks increased during night in the patients with Prinzmetal angina. Was this the natural course or were the patients under intravenous nitroglycerin?

Dr. Chierchia: The patients were all off treatment and they were all in hospital and were allowed to go around the hospital while being monitored with the Holter technique.

Dr. McGregor: The maximum of anginal attacks in the patients with unstable angina was mid-afternoon where one would expect high sympathetic activity.

Dr. Chierchia: Yes, there is clearly a difference between both patient groups and these observations are consistent. We have increased our number of observations considerably. The patients really seem to belong to two different categories.

The patients with classical angina seemed to have a inrual distribution of their attacks, although they may have some ischemic episodes during night as well.

Dr. Bassenge: I completely agree with your general conclusions; however, there were two reports by M. Bertrand, where he was able to resolve spasm in two patients after intracoronary injection of phentolamine. This is quite impressive; how can we explain this?

Dr. Chierchia: The first thing we have to take into account – if I remember correctly – is that Bertrand gave a very large dose of phentolamine in the order of 5 mg intracoronarily, which is a systemic dose. Especially in those high doses phentolamine has been thought to be an unspecific vasodilator. Another possibility would be spontaneous resolution of the spasm.

Dr. Vatner: I don't think that pentholamine is a nonspecific vasodilator. Phentolamine in the presence of ganglionic blockade, increases pressure and is a very potent vasoconstrictor. This is a direct effect of the drug.

Dr. Bassenge: It could be tyramine-like effect, which releases Norepinephrine.

Dr. Chierchia: It should induce ischemia rather then relieve it. Certainly, if you give Phentolamine to some patients with a very low exercise tolerance over a short priod of time, they develop tachycardia and ischemia. Whether ischemia is due to an increase in myocardial oxygen demand in the presence of a very low threshold or possibly related to increased catecholamine release and vasoconstriction or both, I don't know. But certainly in some patients you can induce ischemia by administration of phentolamine in large doses.

Dr. Vatner: I am concerned about the possibility that you may not be blocking the local release of Norepinephrine at the cleft. In other words, with the small doses of blockers you may not abolish agonist-activity.

Dr. Chierchia: We have realized that it is very difficult to manipulate receptors in man. If the alpha-receptors of the epicardial arteries are of the alpha$_2$-type in dog as well as in man, then you can use an alpha$_2$-blocker to block the postsynaptic receptors without preventing blockade of the presynaptic receptors, getting an increased catecholamine release.

Dr. Macilli: You have shown us that at night – and I suppose during sleep – the number of anginal attacks in patients with Prinzmetal angina is much higher. We know that during sleep the sympathetic tone decreases, so please would you comment to the possibility that sympathetic innervation might protect against ischemia attacks?

Dr. Chierchia: To explain that peculiar peak of anginal attacks in the early morning hours, you have many explanations, one was suggested by Dr. Bassenge this morning. If the coronary diameter is smaller because of a lower flow during rest at night and if there is superimposed some bursts of vasoconstrictive stimuli on a smaller diameter to start with, of course the change of getting ischemia is higher. This is one very likely possibility and indeed some Japanese groups have measured coronary artery diameter in the early morning hours, and they found that the coronary diameter was actually smaller. This suggests that there is some circadiane change in the coronary artery diameter.

Dr. Mueller: Cold stimulus increased heart rate by 30% in your patients with variant angina. This appears to be a large increase. In patients with stable angina, cold stimulus induced rise in heart rate is in the order of 10%. Do you think that patients with variant angina have an increased responsiveness?

Dr. Chierchia: They certainly start from a lower point as opposed to patients with chronic stable angina. If you compare two age matched groups of patients with stable angina on one side and variant angina on the other, the variant angina patients start from very low levels of heart rate. Whether this implies a greater reactivity, I don't know.

11. Enhanced transcardiac 1-norepinephrine response during cold pressor test in obstructive coronary artery disease

HILTRUD S. MUELLER, PARINAM S. RAO, PULLIPAKA B. RAO, DENNIS J. GORY, STEPHEN M. AYRES

Introduction

Studies during the past decade have demonstrated that sympathetic nervous activity can play an important role in the regulation of coronary blood flow. It became apparent that alpha adrenergic mediated coronary vasoconstriction can compete with metabolically-induced coronary vasodilatation, particularly in myocardial regions with decreased coronary reserve [1–7]. Recent studies have also emphasized that increased sympathetic nervous activity enhanced ventricular irritability and lowers the threshold to ventricular fibrillation in the ischemic myocardium [8–11]. Since these observations suggest that increases in sympathetic nervous activity could place the patient with obstructive coronary artery disease at increased risk, we measured arterial and coronary sinus 1-norepinephrine contents during relatively mild sympathetic stress in this patient category and compared their response of transcardiac 1-norepinephrine pattern to that in patients with normal coronary arteries. We selected cold pressor stimulation because it is probably similar to the level of sympathetic stress experienced frequently during daily life. Our data indicate that there is a substantially greater increase in coronary sinus 1-norepinephrine concentrations in the patients with obstructive coronary artery disease compared to those without disease.

Methods

Patient selection

Patients, referred to heart catheterization for evaluation of angina pectoris or of atypical chest pain, were eligible for the study if they fulfilled the following criteria: (1) normal cardiac function as judged by clinical findings, chest X-ray and history; (2) no medications except for mild sedative or sublingual nitroglycerin (none 2 h prior to the procedure); (3) no history or findings of hypertension (blood pressure systolic ≥ 150, diastolic ≥ 95 mmHg); (4) age under 70 years.

Kupper, W. (ed.), Coronary tone in ischemic heart disease. ISBN 0-89838-646-2.
© 1984, Martinus Nijhoff Publishers, Boston/The Hague/Dordrecht/Lancaster. Printed in the Netherlands.

116

Procedure and methods

Prior to heart catheterization, the patient was premedicated with diphenhy-
dramine hydrochloride (benadryl), 50 mg i.m. A#8 pigtail catheter was placed
through the femoral artery into the ascending aorta and a #7 Goodale-Lubin
catheter through the femoral vein into the mid portion of the coronary sinus. Left
ventricular and aortic pressures were measured, and aortic and coronary sinus
blood samples obtained. Subsequently, the left hand of the patient, including the
wrist, was immersed into a mixture of water and ice. At the onset of chest pain or
of discomfort of the hand in the icewater or after 2,5 min of cold stimulus without
symptoms, measurements of aortic pressure and sampling of aortic and coronary
sinus blood were repeated. Routine left heart catheterization, including coronary
arteriography, was then performed.

Blood was analyzed for 1-norepinephrine and epinephrine concentrations and
for oxygen tension. Ratios for myocardial 1-norepinephrine uptake (extraction)
or release (production) were calculated by dividing the arterial-coronary sinus
1-norepinephrine difference by the arterial content. Since plasma 1-norepine-
phrine content is the net effect of neuronal 1-norepinephrine release, reuptake
and metabolism (12), the data are referred to as percent myocardial 1-norepine-
phrine 'net uptake' or 'net release'.

Catecholamine contents were determined according to the method of Hallman
et al. (13) using high pressure liquid chromatography, Waters 6000 A, with a LC-4
electrochemical detector. In our laboratory, plasma catecholamine contents of 13
normal volunteers, obtained after 20 min rest in supine position, averaged
168 ± 41 (SD) pg/ml (1-norepinephrine) and 47 ± 17 pg/ml (epinephrine). The
coefficient of variation of 13 duplicate determinations averaged $2.1 \pm 1.5\%$
(1-norepinephrine) and $4.5 \pm 4.2\%$ (epinephrine), respectively. The coefficients
of variation of measurements, obtained at a 10 min interval from patients prior to
heart catheterization in the same environment as the patients, studied, averaged
$7.4 \pm 5.0\%$ and $6.8 \pm 4.9\%$ for 1-norepinephrine in arterial and coronary sinus
blood (n = 30) and $9.2 \pm 5.8\%$ for epinephrine in coronary sinus blood (n = 15).
Data analysis. The response to the cold pressor test within each study group was
tested with a two tailed paired t-test. The difference in responses between the two
study groups was evaluated by analysis of variance baseline values as covariates.
A $p<0.05$ was considered statistically significant.

Results

Patient material

Twenty-three patients (16 males) with normal coronary arteries and 23 patients
(17 males) with abnormal coronary arteries were studied. The age averaged 47

Table 1. Transcardiac catecholamine responses to cold pressor test.

Measurement	Normal coronary arteries (n = 20)			Abnormal coronary arteries (n = 23)			Δ Normal cor. arteries*	Δ Abnormal cor. arteries*	p
	Control*	Cold pressor*	p	Control*	Cold pressor*	p		vs	
Heart rate, beats/min	73 ± 15	80 ± 16	<0.001	76 ± 15	83 ± 22	<0.01	+6.5 ± 7.2	+6.6 ± 11	NS
Arterial pressure, mmHg									
Systolic	138 ± 20	168 ± 26	<0.001	146 ± 20	178 ± 21	<0.001	+29 ± 17	+31 ± 15	NS
Diastolic	78 ± 11	95 ± 13	<0.001	80 ± 10	102 ± 13	<0.001	+17 ± 11	+21 ± 11	NS
Mean	101 ± 13	122 ± 21	<0.001	105 ± 15	132 ± 21	<0.001	+20 ± 16	+27 ± 18	NS
Double product, mmHg × beats/min × 10³	10.3 ± 3.1	13.6 ± 4.0	<0.001	11.2 ± 2.9	14.6 ± 3.6	<0.001	+3.2 ± 2.2	+3.2 ± 1.5	NS
Left ventricular filling pressure, mmHg	10 ± 3.7	–	–	15 ± 4.5	–	–	–	–	–
NE[a] content, pg/ml									
Arterial	295 ± 152	339 ± 174	<0.01	250 ± 134	285 ± 134	NS	+44 ± 67	+ 34 ± 115	NS
Coronary sinus	273 ± 152	301 ± 170	NS	250 ± 115	387 ± 250	<0.002	+28 ± 76	+137 ± 182	<0.012
Myocardial NE net uptake or release, %	7.5 ± 29	10 ± 16	NS	7.2 ± 29	34 ± 53	<0.01	+2.9 ± 25	−27 ± 48	<0.003
EPI[b] content, pg/ml									
Arterial	69 ± 32	76 ± 54	NS	70 ± 43	77 ± 42	NS	+6.5 ± 39	+6.9 ± 29	NS
Coronary sinus	56 ± 29	63 ± 38	NS	60 ± 36	85 ± 53	<0.02	+7.4 ± 21	+25 ± 44	NS

[a] NE = 1-norepinephrine.
[b] EPI = Epinephrine.
* mean ± SD

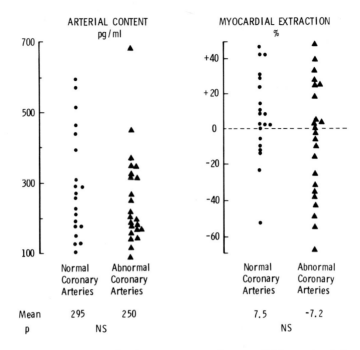

Figure 1. Baseline arterial 1-norepinephrine contents and myocardial 1-norepinephrine ratios. Arterial 1-norepinephrine contents were similar in patients with normal and abnormal coronary arteries. Myocardial 1-norepinephrine net uptake dominanted in patients with normal coronary arteries, while 1-norepinephrine epinephrine net release dominated in those with abnormal coronary arteries.

and 54 years, respectively, ranging from 31 to 65 and 30 to 67 years. The electrocardiogram was normal in all but one of the patients with normal and in ten of the 23 patients with abnormal coronary arteries. Of the patients with coronary artery disease, seven had ≥70% obstruction of one major dominant coronary artery, eight patients of two and eight of three major arteries. One patient had a 70% stenosis of the left main stem. The left ventriculogram was normal in all patients with normal coronary arteries and showed various forms of hypokinesis or akinesis in the patients with disease. During cold stimulus seven of 23 patients with coronary artery disease developed chest pain, associated with ST-segment depression in four and with ST-segment elevation in three. Six patients complained about chest pain without electrocardiographic changes. Two of the 23 patients with normal coronary arteries experienced chest pain without demonstrating other abnormalities.

Data of patients with normal and abnormal coronary arteries

Baseline data of the two patient groups are shown in Table 1 (mean ± SD) and

Figure 1. Heart rate averaged 73 ± 15 and 76 ± 15 beats/min, aortic pressure $138 \pm 20/78 \pm 11$ and $146 \pm 20/80 \pm 10$ mmHg, respectively. The left ventricular end diastolic pressure was the only hemodynamic measurement which differed between the two groups; mean values were 10 ± 3.7 and 15 ± 4.5 mmHg ($p<0.01$). Individual data of arterial 1-norepinephrine contents and of the ratios of myocardial 1-norepinephrine net uptake (extraction) or net release (production) are shown in Figure 1. In all but eight patients plasma 1-norepinephrine contents were below 350 pg/ml (twice the mean value for resting normal volunteers). The myocardial 1-norepinephrine ratios, shown in Figure 1, varied considerably. Two-thirds of the patients with normal coronary arteries demonstrated myocardial 1-norepinephrine net uptake, while more than half of the patients with coronary artery disease showed myocardial 1-norepinephrine net release.

Cold stimulus by insertion of the hand into ice cold water caused changes in hemodynamics which were similar in the patients with normal and abnormal coronary arteries (Table 1, Figure 2). Heart rate increased an average of $10 \pm 11\%$ and $9 \pm 10\%$, respectively, systolic pressure $21 \pm 12\%$ and $22 \pm 13\%$, diastolic presssure $23 \pm 16\%$ and $27 \pm 16\%$, and double product $32 \pm 26\%$ and $29 \pm 16\%$. Increases in arterial 1-norepinephrine contents, like increases in hemodynamic measurements, were similar in both groups, $19 \pm 30\%$ and $26 \pm 58\%$, respectively. In contrast, cold pressor-induced increases in coronary sinus 1-norepinephrine contents differed strikingly, averaging $17 \pm 37\%$ in the normal and $58 \pm 62\%$ in the abnormal coronary artery patients. Accordingly, the myocardial 1-norepinephrine ratios also responded differently to cold stimulus (Figure 3). In

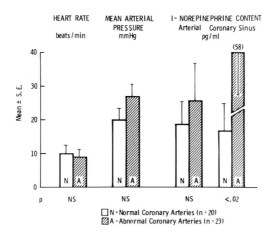

Figure 2. Cold pressor-induced changes in hemodynamics and plasma 1-norepinephrine contents. Average increases in heart rate, mean arterial pressure and arterial 1-norepinephrine contents were similar in patients with normal (open bars) and abnormal (hatched bars) coronary arteries. In contrast, cold pressor-induced increases in coronary sinus 1-norepinephrine contents were three-fold higher in patients with coronary artery disease.

the normal coronary artery group cold stimulus enhanced both percent myocardial 1-norepinephrine net uptake and release; the mean value of the ratios remained essentially unchanged, $7.5 \pm 29\%$ and $10 \pm 16\%$. In the abnormal coronary artery group, however, cold stimulus greatly enhanced percent myocardial 1-norepinephrine net release. Four patients decreased myocardial net uptake and 14 patients shifted from net uptake to release or enhanced 1-norepinephrine net release; the mean value changed from $-7.2 \pm 29\%$ to $-34 \pm 53\%$ ($p<0.01$). 1-Norepinephrine net release was observed in patients with and without findings of myocardial ischemia. Baseline arterial and coronary sinus epinephrine contents averaged about 50% above normal in both patient groups. The response to cold stimulus varied widely, and no statistically significant changes were observed.

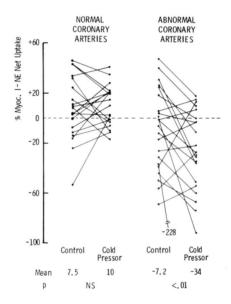

Figure 3. Ratios of myocardial 1-norepinephrine net uptake ($+$) and net 1-norepinephrine release ($-$). At control the majority of patients with normal coronary arteries demonstrated 1-norepinephrine net uptake. The response to cold pressor varied; the mean value remained unchanged. In patients with abnormal coronary arteries myocardial 1-norepinephrine net release dominated at control and was strikingly enhanced during cold stimulus.

Discussion

The appearence of 1-norepinephrine in blood represents a spillover from the synaptic cleft and is dependent upon the level of neural stimulation, neuronal release and reuptake, blood flow and extraneuronal metabolism [12]. Recent studies have suggested that, in spite of these limitations, plasma 1-norepinephrine concentrations may be a better reflection of sympathetic neural activity than formely believed, particularly if 1-norepinephrine contents are measured across one specific organ. Yamaguchi et al. [14] demonstrated a close relationship among myocardial 1-norepinephrine release, coronary blood flow, heart rate and dP/dt during stellate ganglion stimulation in the dog; Cryer et al. [15] showed in man that a prompt increase in heart rate and blood pressure following cigarette smoking was associated with a parallel increase in 1-norepinephrine contents of venous blood.

Transcardiac 1-norepinephrine patterns have been studied under various conditions in man and in the experimental animal. The normal heart extracts 1-norepinephrine under resting conditions [16–29]. 1-Norepinephrine is released by the normal heart under conditions of substantial stress such as rapid cardiac pacing, handgrip exercise [19–21], or stellate ganglion stimulation [14]. The ischemic heart, in contrast, release 1-norepinephrine at rest and this releases may be further increased by the application of certain stresses. Handgrip [19–21] or ergometer exercise [22, 23] leads to enhanced 1-norepinephrine release in patients with coronary artery disease; reperfusion experiments following transient coronary occlusion in experimental animals [24–26] produce similar findings. Remarkably high concentrations of 1-norepinephrine are found in coronary sinus blood in patients with acute myocardial infarction [27].

The present study was designed to determine whether relatively mild stressful stimuli would evoke different responses in individuals with significantly obstructed coronary arteries compared to those with normal coronary arteries. Immersion of the hand in cold water – the classic cold pressor test – was selected as a stimulus that might produce a sympathetic response similar to responses experienced frequently during everyday life.

The transcardiac plasma 1-norepinephrine patterns showed a major difference in the response to cold pressor stimulation between the two patient populations. The mild, balanced increases in the arterial and coronary sinus 1-norepinephrine concentrations in the individuals with normal coronary arteries and normal cardiac function suggest a generalized sympathetic response to afferent stimuli from the periphery [28–30], initiated from the chilled limb. A similar mild increase in arterial 1-norepinephrine concentrations, but a three-fold increase in coronary sinus concentrations in those patients with obstructive coronary artery disease suggest an exaggerated response of the heart. This local cardiac response could reflect a cardio-cardiac reflex as observed by Brown [31, 32] and Malliani [33]. Transient coronary occlusion in the cat resulted in increased discharge of sympathetic afferent and preganglionic nerves associated with an increase in cardiac sympathetic activity. Changes in concentrations of hydrogen ions and potassium, hypoxia and mechanical factors, including myocardial dysfunction [32–35], have been suggested as mechanisms for this reflex. In the present study ischemia and impaired left ventricular function, triggered by cold stimulus, could

122

have evoked a cardio-cardiac reflex. More than half of the patients with significantly obstructed coronary arteries exhibited findings of myocardial ischemia during cold stimulus in form of ST-segment depression, ST-segment elevation and/or angina pectoris. Left ventricular end diastolic pressures were higher in the patients with abnormal coronary arteries compared to those with normal vessels so that cold stimulus-induced increases in blood pressure could have further impaired left ventricular function [7]. This possibility is consitent with the observation in patients with coronary artery disease that myocardial 1-norepinephrine release during handgrip exercise was negatively related to ventricular ejection fraction [20, 21] and that coronary sinus 1-norepinephrine concentrations were positively related to left ventricular end diastolic pressures [36].

Factors other than increase in myocardial release of 1-norepinephrine might have contributed to the rise in coronary sinus 1-norepinephrine concentrations during cold stimulus. 1-Norepinephrine reuptake has been shown to be impaired by myocardial ischemia [37–39]. In addition, cold stimulus-induced decreases of flow in diseased coronary arteries [6, 7] could have exaggerated the rise in coronary sinus 1-norepinephrine concentrations. The design of the study does not allow differentation among the various mechanisms.

The increases in coronary sinus 1-norepinephrine concentrations, observed in our patients with obstructive coronary artery disease during the relatively mild symphathetic stress of cold stimulus, probably occur numerous times during daily routine. Repetitive and cumulative bursts of neurotransmitter could decrease regional coronary perfusion [3–6], increase local oxygen demand [40], change substrate availability [41, 42] and alter electrical properties of the myocardium [8–11]. The potential hazard of increased myocardial 1-norepinephrine concentrations support the suggestion that reducing overall sympathetic tone by anti-adrenergic agents might be a useful therapeutic intervention for patients with ischemic heart disease.

References

1. Murray PA, Vatner SF: Alpha-receptor attenuation of coronary vascular response to severe, spontaneous exercise. Circ Res 45:654–60, 1979.
2. Schwartz PJ, Stone HL: Tonic influence on the sympathetic nervous system on myocardial reactive hyperemia and on coronary blood flow distribution in dogs. Circ Res 41:51–58, 1977.
3. Mohrman DE, Feigl EO: Competition between sympathetic vasoconstriction and metabolic vasodilatation in the canine coronary circulation. Circ Res 42:79–86, 1978.
4. Mudge GH Jr, Grossman W, Mills RM Jr, Lesch M, Braunwald E: Reflex increase in coronary vascular resistance in patients with ischemic heart disease. N Engl J Med 295:1333–1337, 1976.
5. Mudge GH Jr, Goldberg S, Gunther S, Mann T, Grossman W: Comparison of metabolic and vasoconstrictior stimuli on coronary vascular resistance in man. Circulation 59:544–550, 1979.
6. Malacoff RF, Mudge GH Jr, Holman BL, Cohn RF: Effect of the cold pressor test on regional myocardial blood flow in patients with coronary artery disease. Clin Res 28:194A (abstract), 1980.

7. Feldman FL, Whittle JL, Marx JD, Pepine CJ, Conti CR: Regional coronary hemodynamic responses to cold stimulation in patients without variant angina. Am J Cardiol 49:665–673, 1982.

8. Verrier RL, Thompson P, Lown B: Ventricular vulnerability during sympathetic stimulation: Role of heart and blood pressure. Cardiovasc Res 8:602–10, 1974.

9. Kolman B, Verrrier RL, Lown B: The effects of vagus nerve stimulation upon vulnerability during coronary artery occlusion and reperfusion. Circulation 52:578–85, 1974.

10. Corr PB, Gillis RA: Autonomic neural influences on the dysrhythmias resulting from myocardial infarction. Circ Res 43:1–9, 1978.

11. Schwartz PJ, Stone HL: Left stellectomy in the prevention of vetricular fibrillation caused by acute myocardial ischemia in conscious dogs with anterior myocardial infarction. Circulation 62:1256–1265, 1980.

12. Iverson LL: Uptake processes for biogenic amines. In: Iverson LL, Iverson SD, Snyder SH (eds) Handbook of Psychopharmacology. Section 1, Vol 3. Plenum Press, New York, 1975, pp 381–442.

13. Hallman H, Farnebo LO, Hamberger B, Johnson G: Selection method for the determination of plasma cathecholamines using liquid chromatography with electrochemical detection. Life Sci 23:1049–1052, 1978.

14. Yamaguchi N, de Champlain J, Nadeau R: Correlation between the response of the heart to sympathetic stimulation and the release of endogenous catecholamines into the coronary sinus of the dog. Circ Res 36:662–668, 1975.

15. Cryer PE, Haymond MW, Santiago JV, Shah SD: Norepinephrine and epinephrine release and adrenergic mediation of smoking-associated hemodynamic and metabolic events. N Engl J Med 295:573–77, 1976.

16. Raab W, Gigee AB: Specific activity of the heart muscle to absorb and store epinephrine and norepinephrine. Circ Res 3:553–58, 1955.

17. Siegel JH, Gilmore JP, Sarnoff SJ: Myocardial extraction and production of catecholamines. Circ Res 9:1336–1350, 1961.

18. Braunwald E, Harrison DC, Chidsey CA: The heart as an endocrine organ. Am J Med 36:1–4, 1964.

19. Maürer W, Mehmel HC, Zebe H, Opherk D, Müller JH, Kübler W: Freisetzung endogener Katecholamine in den Koronarsinus durch isometric Belastung und frequente Vorhofstimulation bei koronarer Herzkrankheit. Verh Dtsch Ges Kreislaufforschung 42:294–296, 1976.

20. Maürer W, Opherk D, Zebe H, Mehmel HC, Müller JH, Kübler W: Veränderungen des Plasma-Katecholamin-Gehaltes im Koronarsinus bei Patienten mit koronarer Herzerkrankung unter Belastung. Verh Dtsch Ges Inn Med 82: 1193–1196, 1976.

21. Maürer W, Tschada J, Manthey J, Ablasser W, Kübler W: Cathecholamines in patients with heart failure. In: Delius W, Gerlach E, Grobecker H, Kübler W (eds) Catecholamines and the Heart. Springer-Verlag, Berlin, Heidelberg, New York, 1981, pp 236–246.

22. Dominiak P, Schulz W, Kober G, Grobecker H: Simulane Bestimmung von Plasmanoradrenalin in Aorta, peripherer Vene und Koronarvenensinus in Ruhe und unter Belastung. Z Kardiol Suppl 5:73 (abstract), 1978.

23. Delius W, Wirtzfeld A, Dominiak P, Sebening H, Blömer H, Grobecker H: Wirkungen einer akuten Blockade adrenerger β-Receptoren auf Noradrenalinkonzentration und Hämodynamik bei Patienten nach Myokartinfarkt. Z Kardiol 68: 441–448, 1979.

24. Shahab L, Wollenberger A, Haase M, Schiller U: Noradrenalinabgabe aus dem Hundeherzen nach vorübergehender Okklusion einer Koronararterie. Acta Biol Med Germ 22:135–143, 1969.

25. Préda I, Kárpáti P, Endröczi E: Myocardial noradrenaline uptake after coronary occlusion in the rat. Acta Physiol Acad Scient Hungaricae, 46:99–106, 1975.

26. Rochette L, Didier JP, Moreau D, Bralet J: Effect of substrate on release of myocardial norepinephrine and ventricular arrhythmias following reperfusion of the ischemic isolated working rat heart. J Cardiovasc Pharmacol 2:267–279, 1980.

124

27. Mueller HS, Rao PS, Ayres SM: Transcardiac 1-norepinephrine pattern during myocardial infarction in man. Clin Res 30:II–208A (abstract), 1982.
28. Ninomiya I, Nisinaru N, Irisawa H: Sympathetic nerve activity to the spleen, kidney and heart in response to baroreceptor input. Am J Physiol 221:1346–1351, 1971.
29. Kendrick E, Oberg B, Wennergren B: Vasoconstriction fiber discharge to skeletal muscle, kidney, intestine and skin at varying levels of arterial baroreceptor activity in the cat. Acta Physiol Scan 85:464–476, 1972.
30. Hansen JF, Hesse B, Christensen NJ: Enhanced sympathetic nervous activity after intravenous propanolol in ischaemic heart disease: plasma noradrenaline splanchnic blood flow and mixed venous oxygen saturation at rest and during exercise. Eur J Clin Invest 8:31–36, 1978.
31. Brown AM: Excitation of afferent cardiac sympathetic nerve fibers during myocardial ischemia. J Physiol 190:35–53, 1967.
32. Brown AM, Malliani A: Spinal reflexes initiated by coronary receptors. J Physiol 212:685–705, 1971.
33. Malliani A, Schwartz PJ, Zanchetti A: A sympathetic reflex elicited by experimental coronary occlusion. Am J Physiol 217:703–709, 1969.
34. Peterson DF, Brown AM: Pressor reflexes produced by stimulation of afferent fibers in the cardiac sympathetic nerves of the cat. Circ Res 28: 605, 1971.
35. Uchida Y, Murao S: Excitation of afferent cardiac sympathetic nerve fibers during coronary occlusion. Am J Physiol 226:1094–1099, 1974.
36. Hansen JF, Christensen NJ, Hesse B: Determinants of coronary sinus noradrenaline in patients with ischaemic heart disease: coronary sinus catecholamine concentration in relation to arterial catecholamine concentration, pulmonary artery oxygen saturation and left ventricular end-diastolic pressure. Cardiovasc Res 12:415–421, 1978.
37. Sachs C: Noradrenaline uptake mechanisms in the mouse atrium. A biochemical and histochemical study. Acta Physiol Scand 341:1–67, 1970.
38. Schömig A, Dietz R, Rascher W, Strasser R, Kübler W: Noradrenaline release from the ischemic myocardium. Circulation 62 (suppl III):III–176 (abstract), 1980.
39. Dietz R, Schömig A, Strasser R, Kübler W: Catecholamines in myocardial hypoxia and ischemia. In: Delius W, Gerlach E, Grobecker H, Kübler W (eds) Catecholamines and the Heart. Springer-Verlag, Berlin, Heidelberg, New York. 1981, pp 201–209.
40. Newman WH, Mathur PP, Walton RP: Catecholamine and local rebound in left ventricular contractile force after release of coronary artery occlusion. Cardiovasc Res 5:81–85, 1971.
41. Opie LH: Metabolic response during impending myocardial infarction. I. Relevance of studies of glucose and fatty acid metabolism in animals. Circulation 45:483–490, 1972.
42. Mueller HS, Ayres SM: Metabolic responses of the heart in acute myocardial infarction in man. Am J Cardiol 42:363–371, 1978.

Discussion

Dr. Bassenge: There was a considerably higher enddiastolic pressure in the group of patients with coronary heart disease. I wonder, if there were any signs of heart fialure. This would explain part of the results and also indicate that it is important to differentiate where the norepinephrine originates from, either from the vessels or from the myocardium.

Dr. Mueller: Clinically and by chest X-ray, these patients did not show findings or left ventricular fialure. However, the higher enddiastolic pressures in patients with coronary artery disease suggest left ventricular dysfunction. We cannot differentiate whether the stimulus for norepinephrine release came from the myocardium or from the blood vessels. Changes in concentrations of hydrogen ions, potassium and oxygen in ischemic myocardium could have triggered sympathetic stimulation.

Dr. Bassenge: So, if one summarizes it could be that the main release is from the myocardium – from nerve endings within the myocardium.

Dr. Mueller: We do not have information about the site of 1-norepinephrine release. Even under the assumption that 1-noropinephrine release was triggered mainly by ischemic myocardium, this stimulus would exert not only local 1-norepinephrine release from the sympathetic nerve terminal, but also stimulate afferent and efferent sympathetic pathways, resulting in increased 1-norepinephrine release from both, the myocardium and the blood vessels.

Dr. Vatner: The question is, is there a net uptake or increased release?

Dr. Mueller: The design of the study does not allow to differentiate whether there is decreased 1-norepinephrine uptake or increased release. Schömig et al., Circulation 62:III–176, 1980 and other investigators have demonstrated in the experimental animal that myocardial ischemia causes both decreased 1-norepinephrine uptake and increased norepinephrine release.

Dr. Serruys: During the last meeting of the American College of Cardiology a paper was presented entitled: 'Sympathetic nerve acitivity during the cold pressotl test' which was designed very similar to your work, but came to totally different conclusions. They found an arterio-venous (GCV) difference in norepinephrine which was identical in the patients with coronary artery disease and in patients with normal coronary arteries. I wonder if you have any explanation for these differences because they came to the conclusion that probably the reactivity to norepinephrine was different in both groups whereas the levels were similar.

Dr. Mueller: I have no explanation for the differences between the results of our study and those of Dr. D. Reisen (JACC 1:694, 1983). It would be possible that our patients had more severe coronary artery disease.

Dr. Serruys: So, in general, when we are speaking about cold pressor test I think the situation of the patient is really a critical issue because it has been demonstrated this morning that the response to the cold pressor test can differ from group to group and really depends on the severity of the coronary artery disease.

Dr.McGregor: Was there any difference in the O_2-AV-difference across the heart or are there any other indicators that the hearts really became ischemic?

Dr. Mueller: We did not find differences in the arterial-coronary sinus oxygen differences. However in patients with compartments with normal and diseased coronary arteries, it is difficult to detect changes in oxygen contents in mixed coronary sinus blood. Changes are in general small.

Dr. Vatner: It is not surprising to me that you have shown increased norepinphrine release with the cold pressor test in your patients. What is surprising to me that you do not have it in your normals. It is well establishes that, if you stimulate sympathetic nerves to the heart, you are going to get net overflow of catecholamines in the coronary sinus. If you do not see this in your normal patients then you really do not have a very strong sympathetic stimulus.

Dr. Mueller: It is very likely that the response of the individual patient to cold stimulus varied considerably resulting in increased coronary sinus 1-norepine-phrine contents or not. It is difficult to compare cold pressor test in man with sympathetic nerve stimulation in the animal. It was the purpose of the study to choose a *mild* sympathetic stress and demonstrate the difference in response between the patient with normal coronary arteries and with coronary artery disease.

Subject index

A-VO$_2$ difference, 65
Accuracy, 40
Acetylcholine, 50, 55
Active dilation, 64
Adenosine concentration, 68
Adrenergic innervation, 105
Afferent stimuli, 121
Alpha-adrenergic blockade, 80
Alpha-adrenergic receptors, 105
Alpha-adrenergic stimulation, 75, 80
Alpha-adrenergic tone, 1
  unopposed, 2, 67
Alpha-adrenoceptor blockade, 1
Alpha-adrenoceptors, 1
  coronary, 43
Alpha-blockade
  non-selective, 45
  postsynaptic, 47
Alpha$_1$-adrenoceptors, 46
Alpha$_2$-adrenoceptors, 46
Alpha$_2$-blockade, 46
Analysis, geometrical, 15
Angina, exertional, 25
Anginal threshold, 93
Angiographic analysis, quantitative, 26
Angiotensin, 16
Animal preparations, 105
Animals, anesthesized, spinalized, 48
Antagonist, 15
Atenolol, 58
Atherosclerosis, diet induced, 37
Atherosclerotic plaque, 19
Atrial contraction, 73
Atrial waves, 73
Autoinhibition of transmitter release, 54
Autonomic control, 57
Autoregulation, 19

Balloon-pumping, 86
Baroreceptor hypotension, 105
Beta-adrenergic antagonists, 95
Beta-adrenergic mechanisms, 68
Beta-adrenergic receptor stimulation, 60
Beta-adrenergic tone, 2, 57
Beta-adrenoceptors, coronary vascular, 43
Beta-mechanisms, 73
Beta$_1$-adrenergic receptor blockade, 57
Beta$_1$-adrenergic receptors, myocardial, 64
Beta$_1$-adrenergic stimulation, 57
Beta$_2$-adrenergic receptors, vascular, 64
Beta$_2$-receptors, 2
Biopsy, 11
Blockade, muscarinic, 45
Blood flow, pulsatile, 41
Blurring effect, 86

Calcium channel blockers, 55
Calibration, 27
Cardiac transplantation, 89
Cardio-cardiac reflex, 122
Cardioselective beta-blockade, 95
Carotid sinus nerve stimulation, 89
Catecholamine levels, 1
  high, 103
Catecholamine liberation, endogenous, 95
Catecholamine overflow, 109
Catecholamines, circulating, 67
Catheter-tip manometer, 77
Centerline, 27
Cetanserin, 15
Chest pain syndrome, 75
Chest X-ray, 124
Circadiane change, 113
Circumflex coronary dimensions, 61
Cold pressor test, 2, 90, 95, 106, 107, 125
Cold stimulus, 119

Conductance arteries, 1, 43
Conductive vessels, 71
Consequences, hemodynamic, 19
Constriction
   generalized, 16
   neurogenic, 43
   uniform, 11
Constrictor effects, 68
Constrictor influences, neurogenic, 3
Contour positions, 27
Contraction resistance, 20
Coronary A-VO$_2$ difference, 86
Coronary angiography analysis system, 26
Coronary arterial caliber, 77
Coronary arterial diameter, 8
Coronary arterial motion, 86
Coronary arterial spasm, 5
Coronary arteriography, magnified, 77
Coronary artery diameter, 72
Coronary constriction, 43
Coronary constrictor tone, basal, 106
Coronary distending pressure, 82, 106
Coronary occlusion, 72
Coronary oxygen extraction, 44
Coronary regulation, metabolic, 43
Coronary reserve, 115
Coronary resistance, late diastolic, 59
Coronary sinus blood flow, 96
Coronary sinus catecholamines, 91, 108
Coronary sinus O$_2$ content, 65
Coronary sinus thermodilution catheter, 90
Coronary sinus 1-norepinephrine contents,
   115
Coronary smooth muscle, isolated, 49
Coronary spasm, 103
   mechanisms, 43
Coronary tone, 25
Coronary vascular resistance, 2, 81
   late diastolic, 61
   regional, 78
Coronary vasomotor reactivity, 75
Coronary vasomotor tone, 26
Coronary venous oxygen saturation, 45
Curvature analysis, 27

Density, intravascular, 40
Diameter, coronary arterial, 25, 26
Diameter (D)-function, 27
Diameter-resistance relationship, 20
Diffusion gap, 71
Dilatation endothelium mediated, 3
Dilation
   ascending, 50
   endothelium mediated, flow-dependent,
     43, 50

metabolic, 43
Dipyridamole, 55
Double product, 119
Drugs, alpha-adrenolytic, 48
Dynamic coronary obstruction, 14
Dynamic coronary stenoses, 19
Dynamic vascular wall thickening, 30

Efferent sympathetic pathways, 125
Effort angina, 11
Elastic modulus, dynamic incremental, 78
Electromagnetic flow meters, 40
Encroachments, atheromatous luminal, 25
Endothelial cells, 49
Endothelial damage, 3
Endothelial factors, 50
Epicardial artery constriction, 49
Epinephrine, 67, 106
Ergonovine, 3, 8
Ergonovine maleate, 75, 77
Excess flow, 54
Exercise threshold, 112
Extraneuronal metabolism, 120

Fibers, adrenergic, 1
Forearm venous compliance, 107

Geometric theory, 36
Great cardiac vein, 76
Great cardiac venous flow, 79
Grey scales, 41

H-1 receptor stimulation, 37
Handgrip, 106
Handgrip exercise, 121
Heart failure, 124
Heart rate, 67
Heart transplant recipients, 106
Heart transplantation, 1
Histamine, 37
Histochemical studies, 105
Hypercontractility, 15
Hyperemia, reactive, 3, 72
Hyperinflation reflex, 45
Hypersensitivity, 3, 25
Hypokinesis, 118
Hypoxia, luminal, 50

Image intensifier, 27, 77
Indometacin, 53
Intima, thickened, 15
Isolated vessels, 62
Isoprenaline-induced tachycardia, 108
Isoproterenol, 57
Isosorbide dinitrate, 26

Isosorbide dinitrate i.c., 32

Ketanserin, 3
Kinetic energy, 40
Lactate extraction rate, 97

Lactate extraction rate, 97
Lactate production, 100
Lambert-Beer, law, 41
Left ventricular end diastolic pressure, 119
Lesion, eccentric, 11
Ligand binding techniques, 73
Localized spasms, 103

Magnification angiography, 103
Metabolic demands, myocardial, 67
Methergin, 25
Methergin i.v., 32
Methoxamine, 16, 49, 77
Methysergid, 15
Metoprolol, 95
Microvasculature, 87
Miniature gauge, 58
Myocardial contractility, 67
Myocardial ischemia, local, 14
Myocardial metabolic demand, 2
Myocardial oxygen consumption, 93

Neural activation, 68
Neural stimulation, 120
Neuronal release, 120
Neuronal 1-norepinephrine release, 116
Nicotine, 45
Nitroglycerin, 8
Norepinephrine, 43, 67
    neurogenic, 47

Obstruction, idealized, 20
Obstruction diameter, minimal, 30
One-way-acetylation, 54
Optical magnification, 26
Organic lesion, 15
Oxygen extraction, 44
Oxygen uptake, 99

Perfusion pressure, distal, 94
Pericardial fluid, 68, 71
Pericardium, 71
Perivascular nerve stimulation, 49
Persantine, 93
Perspex models, 29
Pharmacologic activation, 68
Phentolamine, 77, 112
Pincushion distortion, 27
Pirbuterol, 57

Pitressin, 16
Plasma catecholamine levels, 107
Plasma catecholamines, 46
Pliability, 38
Posterior hypothalamus, 105
Poiseuille's law, 19
Prazosin, 58, 109
Prenalterol, 57, 58, 64
Pressure, distending, 16, 40
Pressure drop, 19
Pressure gradient, 20
Pressure-diameter relationship, 77
Prinzmetal angina, 103
Propranolol, 58, 65
Prostacycline, 53
Provocative testing, 108
PTCA, 41
Pulmonary inflation reflex, 45
Pulmonary pressures, 96
Pulsatile diameter changes, 86
Pulse diameter, 78
Pulse pressure, 78

QT interval, 107

Rapid cardiac pacing, 121
Rauwolscine, 94
Reaction, hypocontractile, 15
Reactive hyperemia, 68
Receptors, muscarinic cholinergic, 106
Reference diameter, luminal, 30
Reflex withdrawal, 45
Reflexes, 44
    activation, 44
Reninangiotensin system, 46
Resistance vessels, 1, 2, 43

Serotonine, 55
Serotonin antagonists, 3
Serumlactate, 96
Shear stress, 43, 50
Signal, dilatory, 50
Smooth muscle, 11
Spasm
    catheter-induced, 11
    ergonovine-induced, 5
    exercise-induced, 107
    spontaneous resolution, 113
ST-segment depression, 101
ST-segment elevation, 106
Stellate ganglion activity, 107
Stellate ganglion stimulation, 121
Stenosis
    eccentric, 38
    fixed, 103

organic, 5
Stenotic lesions, collapsing, 40
Sympathectomy, chemical, 54
Sympathetic coronary innervation, 43
Sympathetic fibres, 105
Sympathetic stimulation, 1
Sympathetic tone, resting, 72
Synaptic cleft, 120

Tone
    constrictor, 1
    smooth muscle, 21
Tortion movement, 86
Total peripheral resistance, 76
Transcardiac 1-norepinephrine pattern, 115
Transmitter release, 46
Treadmill exercise, 11
Trimazosin, 91

Ultrasonic dimension gauge, 58
Ultrasonic signal, 58
Ultrasonic transducers, 57

Vagal withdrawal, 64
Variant angina, 5, 95
    autopsied, 6
Vascular reactivity, 57
Vascular wall distensibility, 78
Vascular wall thickening, dynamic, 29

Vasoconstriction
    alpha-adrenergic, 1
    upstream, 93
    variable, 19
Vasoconstrictor response, 90
Vasoconstrictor stimuli, 21
Vasodilation, 2
Vasodilatory reserve, 101
Vasomotion, 33
Vasomotor reactivity, 11, 14
Vasomotor tone, 15, 33
    inappropriate, 3
Vasospasm
    coronary, 1
    exercise-induced, 1
    spontaneous, 15
Vasospastic angina, 107
Vasospastic angina mechanism, 2
Vasotonic angina, 14
Ventricle, non-working, 50
Ventricular fibrillation, 3, 115
Ventricular irritability, 3
Vessel, normal segments, 16
Viscosity, 19

Walk through angina, 56
Wall area, 36

Xenon, 87, 133